Caring for Our Communities

Caring for Our Communities

Communities

A Blueprint for Better Outcomes in Population Health

Mark Angelo, MD

Foreword by David B. Nash, MD, MBA

ACHE Management Series

Your board, staff, or clients may also benefit from this book's insight. For information on quantity discounts, contact the Health Administration Press Marketing Manager at (312) 424-9450.

This publication is intended to provide accurate and authoritative information in regard to the subject matter covered. It is sold, or otherwise provided, with the understanding that the publisher is not engaged in rendering professional services. If professional advice or other expert assistance is required, the services of a competent professional should be sought.

The statements and opinions contained in this book are strictly those of the author and do not represent the official positions of the American College of Healthcare Executives or the Foundation of the American College of Healthcare Executives.

Library of Congress Cataloging-in-Publication Data
Names: Angelo, Mark (Palliative medicine physician), author. | American College of Healthcare Executives, issuing body.
Title: Caring for our communities : a blueprint for better outcomes in population health / Mark Angelo.
Other titles: Management series (Ann Arbor, Mich.)
Description: Chicago, IL : Health Administration Press, [2023] | Series: ACHE management series | Includes bibliographical references and index. | Summary: "There has never been a more compelling time to adopt a system of care based on population health management. The COVID-19 pandemic revealed substantial health disparities. The population is aging, and the Medicare insolvency crisis is looming. Now is the time to move away from fee-for-service care and toward an approach that prioritizes quality, outcomes, and affordability for all populations. In Caring for Our Communities: A Blueprint for Better Outcomes in Population Health, author Mark Angelo shares the expertise he has acquired as a senior administrator of a large accountable care organization and a leader in population health and palliative medicine. He provides tactical guidance for developing effective population health programs and explores value-based care models. He also uses real-world examples and industry experts' views to clarify the concepts underlying value-based initiatives and shares how data and analytics are used to assess the health and needs of a population. Caring for Our Communities provides a road map for creating an equitable, outcomes-focused system, using the right resources to nurture the health of our communities"–Provided by publisher.
Identifiers: LCCN 2023034491 | ISBN 9781640554269 (trade paperback ; alk. paper) | ISBN 9781640554276 (ebook) | ISBN 9781640554283 (epub)
Subjects: MESH: Community Health Services–organization & administration | Population Health | Accountable Care Organizations–organization & administration | Value-Based Health Care–organization & administration | United States
Classification: LCC HB883.5 | NLM WA 546 AA1 | DDC 363.9–dc23/eng/20230908
LC record available at https://lccn.loc.gov/2023034491

ISBN: 978-1-64055-426-9

The paper used in this publication meets the minimum requirements of American National Standard for Information Sciences—Permanence of Paper for Printed Library Materials, ANSI Z39.48-1984. ∞™

Manuscript editor: Kevin McLenithan; Cover designer: Mark Oberkrom; Layout: Integra

Found an error or a typo? We want to know! Please e-mail it to hapbooks@ache.org, mentioning the book's title and putting "Book Error" in the subject line.

For photocopying and copyright information, please contact Copyright Clearance Center at www.copyright.com or at (978) 750-8400.

Health Administration Press
A division of the Foundation of the American
   College of Healthcare Executives
300 S. Riverside Plaza, Suite 1900
Chicago, IL 60606-6698
(312) 424-2800

To my family and to all the strong women in my life who have helped me succeed, especially my mother, my wife, and my daughter. Thank you for all the love and support.

Contents

Foreword   ix

Preface   xv

Acknowledgments   xxiii

Chapter 1.   Perverse Incentives   1

Chapter 2.   Population Health: The Infinite Game   11

Chapter 3.   Community Wellness: The Promise of More
             Equitable Outcomes   27

Chapter 4.   Accountable Care Organizations   43

Chapter 5.   Payviders: Symbiosis to Drive Value-Based
             Care   57

Chapter 6.   Intensive Analytics   71

Chapter 7.   Behavioral Health and Palliative Care:
             Uncovering Unmet Needs   89

Chapter 8.   Improving Coordination and Management
             Along the Continuum of Care   109

Chapter 9.   Building Platforms for Population Health   133

Chapter 10. Into the Future of Value-Based Care   151

Index   167
About the Author   181

Foreword

By David B. Nash, MD, MBA

WE IN THE US healthcare system have been striving for a long time toward what lies in store for you in this book.

It was late November 1999 when the Institute of Medicine (IOM) released the findings of its report titled *To Err Is Human: Building a Safer Health System*. It slammed all of us—not just healthcare professionals, but everyone—into the reality that anywhere from 44,000 to 98,000 people were dying in this country every year from preventable medical errors (Kohn, Corrigan, and Donaldson 2000). Less than two years later, the IOM's Committee on Quality of Health Care in America followed up with *Crossing the Quality Chasm: A New Health System for the 21st Century*, which was intended to provide us with a roadmap for creating that new system.

With its six aims, or domains, of healthcare quality—safe, timely, effective, efficient, equitable, and patient-centered (or STEEEP) care—*Crossing the Quality Chasm* began what I sometimes think of as the first of three waves of a movement in healthcare. It laid out for us the characteristics that care of the future would need (IOM 2001).

The second wave came in 2008 with "The Triple Aim: Care, Health, and Cost" by Berwick, Nolan, and Whittington. Page 1 of this paper laid out the purpose of this new model: "Improving the U.S. health care system requires simultaneous pursuit of three aims: improving the experience of care, improving the health of populations, and reducing per capita costs of health care." This second wave was capped off in dramatic fashion in 2010 with the passage of the Patient Protection and Affordable Care Act, or Obamacare.

In 2020 the third wave—the coronavirus pandemic—crashed upon us, exposing grave shortcomings in our healthcare system and punctuating wide-ranging failures in all of the domains of care that were identified in the first wave of the movement, perhaps especially the domain of healthcare equitability.

In late 2022 I released a book with Charles Wohlforth titled *How Covid Crashed the System: A Guide to Fixing American Health Care*. In the introduction of the book, Sandro Galea, MD, DrPh—dean of the Boston University School of Public Health—noted that it was not until chapter 6 of the book that we started examining hospitals, "because the health system is so much larger than the medical industry." He concluded with what could be called the spirit of the third wave of the movement: "The health system is the entire complex of our life conditions that determine our health. In the wake of this unimaginable tragedy, we must look closely and critically at this system as a whole and find the path to a healthier and more resilient society" (Nash and Wohlforth 2022, 4).

That spirit is carried forward in the pages of Mark Angelo's *Caring for Our Communities*. If *Crossing the Quality Chasm* was the parent of what we are striving for in healthcare, then this book could be considered a child of that movement. When I first read the early outline and sample chapters of this book, I thought, *This is the next level, 3.0, the next generation's voice.* And then the question in my mind became *Will this be the generation that will operationalize what we have been talking about since even before 1999?*

RIDING THE WAVES WITH DR. ANGELO

My professional connection with Mark began in 2014, when he was working in Camden, New Jersey, at Cooper University Health System as a leader in palliative medicine and population health.

Mark reached out to me and other members of the Jefferson College of Population Health as he was starting up an accountable
care organization (ACO) and working to improve the care of the
community in New Jersey. Mark impressed me with his dedication
to his community and to helping improve the quality of care for
patients in the region.

I later got to work more closely with Mark when he joined the
Delaware Valley Accountable Care Organization (DVACO), which
is part of Jefferson Health. Mark joined as the chief medical officer
and was quickly moved into the chief executive officer (CEO) seat
with the surprise resignation of the prior CEO. I was fortunate to be
a board member of DVACO at that time, and Mark and I worked
together closely to help build a strong and viable clinical strategy
and advance the mission of population health.

Mark is a tremendous leader who served during a very tumultuous time in healthcare, both at the ground level in Philadelphia and
in a greater role for the ACO movement. He excels as a diplomat,
which was a big plus in the organization because of its complicated
governance structure. At the time, DVACO had two health system
owners, which is quite out of the ordinary, especially since the owners were also friendly competitors.

Leading DVACO was a challenge, made even more complicated
when Mark facilitated the creation of a joint venture with Humana,
a long-established Fortune 100 healthcare company with great experience in the Medicare Advantage space. This was the first time that
Humana had controlled an ACO of this caliber. Mark was able to
engage all parties with a team of talented individuals to reach common ground on contract terms as well as an aggressive yet viable
strategic business plan.

My role in collaborating with Mark was unique, especially in
the Humana joint venture transaction, because I helped maintain
frank but respectful conversation among the three parties as Humana
went into this new territory with the purchase of the ACO. With
Mark's help, and largely behind the scenes, we kept everybody on
the straight and narrow path during the two years of diplomacy that

brought this to fruition. As a result, these efforts were successful in creating an effective payer–provider relationship that has proven successful even early in its endeavors.

REENGINEERING THE PAYER–PROVIDER RELATIONSHIP

I believe ACOs are evolving, but not fast enough on their own. DVACO represents the next generation of ACOs under a quirky term—the "payvider"—which is hard for people to get their heads around. In my latest book, as in this one by Mark, an entire chapter is devoted to the payvider. DVACO could be the poster child for what the payvider of the future looks like, and I think the Humana/DVACO deal is a part of that powerful trend. There will undoubtedly be different models in the future. They may involve joint ventures, complete ownership, or all kinds of arrangements we're not yet aware of, but I believe this is a critically important national trend. This book answers many of the questions surrounding payvider and ACO models, and it does so through the lens of our post-pandemic realities in managing population health and community wellness.

This book addresses many different arenas in healthcare. It is like a chameleon, taking on different colors depending on your perspective. It will fit comfortably in the classroom and in the boardroom. If you are a hardcore hospital person, the book is highly relevant because you would not understand most of the vocabulary of population health without it. If you are an insurer or managed care–only person, this book is valuable because you might not know the value-based provider vocabulary. The book truly serves as a roadmap of how we think about population health and how we create successful programs to manage accountable care.

In the arc of our work, we have a major post-pandemic opportunity, and *Caring for Our Communities* fits perfectly, tapping into its needs. There is already an entire genre of pandemic-related books from the likes of Shantanu Nundy (*Care After Covid*), Andy Slavitt (*Preventable*), and Nicholas Christakis (*Apollo's Arrow*).

This book is not that.

Caring for Our Communities is the post-pandemic world. The pandemic stunned us with how deep the relationship between population health and equitable care goes. A full chapter of this book is devoted to health equity specifically, but equitable care is a winding thread throughout. Health equity forms the foundation of our third wave but is a frontier we have only begun to cross. *Caring for Our Communities* shows us why this is perhaps the most valuable lesson the pandemic has taught us.

Health equity was never before in the forefront as it is today. Frankly, during the past three decades, I *thought* we were talking about equity, never nearly as much as we needed to. Health equity is a special challenge, and I believe this book is going to contribute to its prominence in the current conversation.

What we don't need at this point in our third wave is another conversation on, for example, whether we should have a national health system. That is all a distraction in an industry where critical issues need to be tackled now. What we need is a road map—a guide with pragmatic advice provided by a compassionate and highly competent leader in the field with proven results. Nuts and bolts.

This book is that.

A board-certified internist, Dr. David B. Nash is internationally recognized for his work in public accountability for outcomes, physician leadership development, and quality-of-care improvement. For more than a decade he has served as a member of the board of directors for Humana, Inc., one of the nation's largest publicly traded healthcare companies. At the Jefferson College of Population Health, Dr. Nash is the founding dean emeritus and remains on the full-time faculty as the Dr. Raymond C. and Doris N. Grandon Professor of Health Policy. He has served for more than 30 years on the university faculty. Repeatedly named to Modern Healthcare's *list of most powerful persons in healthcare, his national activities cover a wide scope.*

REFERENCES

Berwick, D. M., T. W. Nolan, and J. Whittington. 2008. "The Triple Aim: Care, Health, and Cost." *Health Affairs* 27(3): 759–69. https://doi.org/10.1377/hlthaff.27.3.759.

Institute of Medicine (IOM). 2001. *Crossing the Quality Chasm: A New Health System for the 21st Century*. Washington, DC: National Academy Press.

Kohn, L. J., J. M. Corrigan, and M. S. Donaldson (eds.). 2000. *To Err Is Human: Building a Safer Health System*. Washington, DC: National Academy Press.

Nash, D. B., and C. Wohlforth. 2022. *How COVID Crashed the System: A Guide to Fixing American Health Care*. Lanham, MD: Rowman & Littlefield.

Preface: Making the Right Thing to Do the Easy Thing to Do

People are dying because we can't communicate in ways that allow us to understand one another.

Alan Alda

BY ITS NATURE, healthcare is complicated, but explaining to someone what we are trying to accomplish is even more difficult. Still, it is critical that we make it clear. It is literally a matter of life and death, as Alan Alda states above in his 2017 book on relating and communicating, which is delightfully titled *If I Understood You, Would I Have This Look on My Face?*

Alda emphasizes that he is not exaggerating and then adds, "When patients can't relate to their doctors and don't follow their orders, when engineers can't convince a town that the dam could break, when a parent can't win the trust of a child enough to warn her off a lethal drug, they can all be headed for a serious ending" (Alda 2017, xiii).

I can tell you from experience that this statement from someone who played a fictional TV doctor is not hyperbole. As providers in healthcare, we often do a fair job of telling our patients what we want them to do for us. In fact, a lot of medical care has been designed around telling patients what to do. Where providers tend to fall short is in listening, understanding the barriers to good health outcomes, and helping patients reach those better outcomes.

That is why I wrote this book: to explore the importance of managing a population and helping our communities achieve the best outcomes possible. Achieving these goals takes partnerships—with our physicians and other providers, with patients, with communities, and with resources to mitigate barriers to care.

I'm not going to sugarcoat it: there is still a lot of work to be done.

As you will see from the beginning of the first chapter, healthcare professionals and consumers of healthcare alike have long been at the mercy of a system that incentivizes behavior that does not support the health of communities or the goal of managing people to wellness. Its voracious appetite for fee-for-service revenue has driven the US healthcare system toward inequity, extremely high cost, and diminishing outcomes.

I wrote this book not only for people in our communities but also for healthcare leaders, legislators, civic leaders, and people coming up in the health professions as well. The work of healthcare is all-consuming for those of us who care for patients, and evolving the paradigm of care adds yet another level of challenge. We should not be adding yet another task to the plates of our providers in the examination room with their patients. To succeed, we must create and support collaborative systems that *make the right thing to do the easy thing to do* in our healthcare system. There is nothing easy about that charge.

At the time of this writing, I am president and CEO of a large accountable care organization that holds successful risk contracts with multiple payers. It includes a large and highly complex Medicare Shared Savings Program population and multiple commercial and Medicare Advantage programs that serve the communities of southeastern Pennsylvania and southern New Jersey. Still, my roots are solidly planted in internal medicine and palliative medicine, and I continue to regularly practice.

I entered the world of palliative care after several years of practice as an internist. My journey was somewhat unique in that I had the opportunity to be a primary care physician with a large and busy practice within an integrated healthcare delivery system while also doing hospital-based work, seeing inpatients through their stays. As the fields have evolved over the subsequent years, it has become rare now for one physician to have the opportunity to deliver both inpatient and outpatient care, especially in the physician-dense greater metropolitan areas. I consider myself fortunate for having that experience and gaining the perspectives that come along with it.

My internal medicine practice also gave me the opportunity to be the medical director for an area hospice. Yes, my days were long and usually a bit hectic, but I loved the opportunity to be part of a comprehensive care team focused on the management of individuals. This drew me to the field of hospice and palliative medicine, where I pursued my second board certification.

My hospice and palliative care certification gave me the chops to start a comprehensive palliative service at Cooper University Health Care in Camden, New Jersey. Since the specialty of palliative medicine was so new and reimbursement for those services was so challenging, starting a new program was the biggest trial of my career at the time. Through some sweat equity, relationship building, and a super-smart team, we built a strong and sustainable program that put palliative care at the forefront in our region.

As a palliative care physician, I always knew I had the best job in the health system. I had the opportunity to meet so many interesting people and families who were confronting the gravest challenges of human existence. Our practice saw patients who experienced chronic illness or who suffered with years of medications, hospitalizations, surgeries, rehabilitation, and even chemotherapy. At times, we encountered people dealt a devastating illness who were working to regain their composure in their new "self plus illness" persona. Through their challenges, I have been awed by the fortitude these people displayed to keep moving forward in their journeys. I remain in awe of their adaptability, in awe of how these individuals pivot their lives from the typical work–family–sleep cycle to being a patient, which interrupts all aspects of that now-coveted routine.

Not only did I get to meet a host of stimulating yet battle-tested individuals; I got to treat a host of pain and other symptoms through various levels of pathophysiology. My charge was to make people feel better so they could continue with a course of treatment most consistent with their goals. Feeling better does not always happen through drugs. Sometimes, feeling better requires a solid approach to active listening. Sometimes it involves sitting quietly while an individual unveils their issues with their medical care, their family, or the outright betrayal by their body, which is failing them as we sit together.

Practicing palliative care has allowed me to focus on those things that matter most to patients: mobility, independence, symptom control, emotional well-being, and individual preferences for care. It opened my eyes to look beyond my meaning of the word "outcome" to theirs, which can be profoundly deep yet simple at the same time.

To say that the practice of palliative medicine gives a doctor perspective on life is the understatement of my lifetime. While it may seem that many years of managing serious illness can make one callous to the struggles of the individual, my experience has been quite the opposite. For that, I am most fortunate.

On one anniversary of starting the palliative service, I sat back and reflected upon how many lives our nurse Barbara and I had the opportunity to affect over the years. We spoke about how the care and wraparound services offered to the seriously ill population were delivered so late in life: "If only we could extend those services to the left of the lifeline." Thus was conceived my career in population health.

In this book you will learn how population health involves the management of the wellness of a population across many different areas. You will hear stories of successes and challenges for individual patients as well as for populations. You will learn how moving from the legacy model of fee-for-service care delivery to a new paradigm of care that focuses on quality outcomes is beneficial to patients, physicians, and the health system in general.

The population health approach is not a particularly new one. It has been around for years, with some fits and starts when it comes to implementation. Population health was boosted by the Affordable Care Act of 2010 and further advanced by the bipartisan Medicare Access and CHIP Reauthorization Act of 2015. Many health insurance consumers are already part of a value-based arrangement and are just not aware of that. Unfortunately, for a host of reasons, we providers and healthcare leaders have not informed and educated our constituents very well about the importance of getting value in their care.

WHAT LIES AHEAD IN CARING FOR OUR COMMUNITIES

In chapter 1, you will learn about the current and historical challenges to the healthcare delivery system, especially as it relates to cost and provider incentives. Chapter 2 dives into the principles of population health while demonstrating methods for how a system can focus on maintaining wellness for a population, all while still remaining financially viable.

Chapter 3 moves into an in-depth discussion of health equity. In particular, this chapter explains why health equity is important and must be the focus for any successful value-based care approach.

Chapter 4 describes accountable care organizations (ACOs), along with their structure and their function of providing high-quality and high-value outcomes to a large population.

Chapter 5 explores the new "payvider" model of care delivery with close collaboration between payers and providers to deliver on the mission of superior outcomes for patients. Next, chapter 6 discusses the use of intensive analytics for the purpose of providing an essential, deeper look into the population for which providers are responsible. The value-based care model of care delivery is highly dependent on being able to synthesize understanding of our populations from multiple sources transparently.

Chapter 7 moves into a discussion of the essential aspects of care for managing populations, including behavioral health and palliative care. Chapter 8 continues that journey, describing how we use care coordination to manage patients with chronic illness and to strive toward a wellness model for the population.

Chapter 9 describes a tactical blueprint for creating population health management systems to usher in the new, sustainable model of high-quality, accountable care. And finally, chapter 10 outlines some of the challenges to this model of care delivery and presents what is on tap for the future of value-based care through interviews with several visionary thought leaders.

As we get started, we should review a few important definitions to prepare you for the pages to come.

- When I refer to "physicians" in this book, I mean medical doctors in the practice of allopathic or osteopathic medicine. Much of what I am referring to can be translated to other types of doctors, but that is not the primary intent.

- Also, the term "providers," while often used interchangeably with "physicians" in common parlance, is meant to refer to the larger body of providers who are licensed to deliver independent medical care. This would include physicians as well as advanced practice providers such as nurse practitioners and physician assistants.

- Population health is fueled by the value-based care payment system, and the terms are often used synonymously. My interview subjects and I will do the same throughout this book.

- Since primary care is the typical entry point for patients and is so ubiquitous in the realm of medical care, this book will focus on primary care and how models of primary care can be shaped to improve the health of the community. Several of the aspects of value-based care can be translated to specialty care delivery, but the tactics may not be the same.

- ACOs can take on many different shapes based on the needs of their beneficiaries. Some may focus on a

Medicaid population, while others focus on Medicare or commercial insurance recipients. Since the populations are different, the strategies for success may differ. For ease of explanation, I use some generalizations in this book.

- Patient confidentiality is crucial to me. All patient names in the stories you are about to read have been changed to protect their anonymity. Some cases have had some details changed to further protect patient confidentiality.

While I have experienced many of the benefits of a population health approach, I strive throughout this book to present a balanced perspective on the benefits and challenges of this approach to care delivery. You will read in chapters 9 and 10 that significant infrastructure still needs to be built and honed to create true value for our patients.

I have had the opportunity in my career to train many exceptional young physicians, including medical students, residents, fellows, and even attending physicians. One overarching theme that I share with physicians is equally germane to this book. Many providers who have worked with me have heard me give the following advice:

Someday you will need to access the health system, perhaps as a scared patient looking up from a stretcher, a worried parent holding your child's hand, or a grieving son or daughter. If you practice with integrity in all interactions with your patients, you will experience the same in return. Contribute to a system that cares for others and not solely for the purpose of maximizing revenue, and that system you helped build will give you the integrity that you deserve as well.

Finally, please allow me to thank you, the reader of this book. I hope you find it interesting and inspiring. Mostly, I hope that through this conversation, together we will fuel the flames of transformation to improve the health of our communities on a grand scale.

REFERENCE

Alda, A. 2017. *If I Understood You, Would I Have This Look on My Face?: My Adventures in the Art and Science of Relating and Communicating*. New York: Random House.

Acknowledgments

THIS BOOK WOULD not be possible without the expertise and guidance of my editor, Lee Reeder. Thank you, Lee, for being my guide through this process.

Special thanks to the leadership and population health teams at Delaware Valley ACO as well as Jefferson Health, Main Line Health, and Humana.

A very special thank you also goes to my contributors and subject matter experts:

- Dr. David Nash
- AbsoluteCare leaders Dr. Greg Foti and Dr. Anoop Raman
- Aneesh Chopra
- Dr. Cori McMahon
- Dr. Catherine Pantik
- Tony Reed
- George Renaudin
- Dr. David Shulkin

CHAPTER 1

Perverse Incentives

It is difficult to get a man to understand something when his salary depends upon his not understanding it.
Upton Sinclair (1934)

A TALE OF TWO SARAS

It is Friday—the last day of the workweek and a mild fall day with a beautiful weekend on the horizon. But this Friday will be neither a workday nor a nice day for Sara. Unfortunately, Sara has contracted a particularly nasty stomach virus, which has left her hovering constantly between the bedroom and the bathroom. For almost 18 hours, she has been unable to keep anything down. She sits at home, wishing that her stomach could settle down a little, waiting to go out and get some Pedialyte because she is feeling dehydrated.

Sara calls her doctor's office for advice. Unfortunately, they can't get her in today, and the doctor is not available to talk at the moment. Upon recognizing that Sara is a diabetic, the nurse tells her to go to the nearest emergency department (ED), where they will give her intravenous (IV) fluids for hydration and some antiemetic medication to calm the gastrointestinal issues. On that advice, she heads for the hospital. Upon arrival, she is unable to walk into the waiting area and approaches the podium set up outside, where a nurse is signing people in. Sara is directed to take a seat in a group of folding chairs outside. Busy day in the ED, apparently.

After nearly four hours of waiting, Sara is now in a chair in a hallway full of gurneys inside the ED. She quietly sits among patients with a wide range of issues from obvious trauma to colds or flu. Some seem to be unconscious and are hooked up to multiple monitors. Sara hates the sight of blood, and that is not helping her gut. She is starting to feel thirsty but is afraid that her gurgling stomach will come springing to life again if she tries to get some water down. She asks a passerby for some chips of ice, but he is a paramedic heading back to his ambulance and cannot help.

In the hustle and bustle of the busy Friday afternoon in the ED, Sara tries to flag someone down who resembles the person who signed her in and took her vitals. Maybe that person is in charge of her case. The patient in the chair next to Sara is not looking well at all. He starts forcefully coughing and wheezing. Then he starts sneezing. Sara quickly stands up, trying to find another chair a little farther away, and she passes out.

When she comes to, Sara finds herself on a stretcher, and the staff is at long last getting that IV in her arm. Unfortunately, the technician is also bandaging the back of her head, which apparently broke her fall on the corner of a crash cart. She is told that she'll need to have a few tests on her heart and to stay in the hospital overnight. With a sore head and sour stomach, Sara wonders how much will be done in the hospital on the verge of the weekend and whether she will only "stay overnight."

What an ordeal. Did it have to be?

Let us rewind this scenario several hours to look at another outcome. Sara calls her doctor's office for advice on her gastrointestinal illness. Recognizing that Sara is diabetic, the nurse asks, "Are you feeling well enough to drive?" Sara is not so sure about that, so the nurse arranges for transportation to the office. Upon arrival, a staff member takes Sara back into an examination room where she is given antiemetics by mouth for nausea and some fluids to drink. Sara starts drinking with some hesitancy until she can be sure her body won't reject the fluids. It takes about an hour, but she finds she is able to keep more down. The medical assistant checks her blood sugar and gives her some crackers to further test her gut.

Ninety minutes later, Sara sits in an Uber on her way home with instructions from her physician. She stops at the store for some Pedialyte to continue her hydration and then heads home, looking forward to a well-deserved nap. Nobody coughing in her face, no bandage on her head, no waiting for a hospital bed on a gurney in the ED, and no ED or hospital charges to contend with.

Which of those two scenarios would you rather experience as a patient? Need I ask?

How does our healthcare delivery system move on from a paradigm where the path of least value to the patient is the default answer? How do we get from the first scenario—long ED wait times, sequelae of dehydration, unwanted workups—to that second, more favorable experience? How do we make the right thing to do in healthcare the easy thing to do? The answer to that last question is a major theme that we will discuss in depth throughout this book.

To start, let's first consider what brings us to this point in our medical care delivery.

How do we make the right thing to do in healthcare the easy thing to do?

ALTRUISM MEETS TRUISMS

The overwhelming majority of medical students go into medicine with altruistic intentions. I cannot tell you how many times I have heard about the desire to help people, cure disease, bring comfort to the sick, and make a positive impact on society. Graduating medical students bring this satchel of good intentions with them into practice, but somewhere between graduation and completion of formal training, those intentions meet reality.

When residency training is behind them, newly minted doctors meet the realities of what it takes to make a medical practice succeed. Long hours and short visits are accompanied by payment struggles, documentation requirements, and insurance quibbles. Rookie physicians are compelled to create a new mental model for practice in a way that delivers top-notch care and outcomes while maintaining a new focus on the business of medicine. That is the time when physicians learn to keep another spinning plate in motion: building and sustaining a career in medical practice.

UNDERSTANDING MEDICAL PRACTICES IN AMERICA

There are multiple types of medical practices out there. Increasingly common now are the large employed medical groups. These practices may be owned and managed by health systems, health insurers, or even for-profit venture capital firms. These groups often pay their providers a flat salary or some variable pay based on some measure of productivity. Productivity measures may include the size of the provider's panel or—more commonly—revenue generated directly through patient encounters. Typical salaries for providers in employed groups include incentives to complete tasks that the practice may be expected to deliver. Incentives can be pretty much anything under the sun: completion of documentation in a timely manner, willingness to accept new patients, nontraditional office hours, quality goal achievement, or even patient experience and ratings. The list of potential incented behaviors is long and varies depending on the priorities of the practice.

Outside of employed medical groups, there are independent practices. While some of these independent practices operate on multisite or even multistate delivery models, independent practices tend to be smaller than health systems or insurer employed practices and are reminiscent of the old-fashioned "hang out a shingle" practices. Independent practices have made exceptional strides in sophistication over the years. These providers tend to be charismatic and highly motivated to succeed in delivering sound, personalized medical care with a strong business plan backing them up. Reimbursement for these providers is often based on patient revenue.

Unfortunately, in the wake of multiple waves of COVID and subsequent economic struggles, many independent providers have seen a significant bite taken out of their revenue. Expense challenges include stagnant reimbursement in the setting of skyrocketing costs for staff, billing, and vital supply chain items. To combat stagnant revenue and rising expenses, practices are left scrambling for new methods of increasing patient revenue. Providers may elect to see additional patients throughout the week or take on new activities, such as bariatric practice or minor cosmetic procedures.

Given the stress of the pandemic on providers and resources, by the end of 2020 nearly 50,000 physicians left independent medical practice to become employees of hospitals or other corporate entities. That represents a 12 percent increase in employed providers, resulting in nearly 75 percent of all physicians in America practicing under the employment of health systems or other corporately owned practices such as private equity or health insurers (Physicians Advocacy Institute 2022).

BEHAVIORAL ECONOMICS FOR PHYSICIANS

Medical encounters across America have historically been geared toward *telling patients what to do*, and the reimbursement system has historically supported doctors in this journey. *Don't smoke. Take your medications. Don't eat trans fats. Start a fitness regimen.* The final outcomes of these efforts to tell patients what to do did not particularly matter for reimbursement. What mattered more was to document that doctors told the patient what to do, including the time involved in doing so. If the patient didn't follow physician instructions, it was somehow less relevant. There was simply no way to measure the nuances of those conversations, leaving only "good patients" and "noncompliant patients."

This is a good point to mention that the overwhelming majority of physicians I have met in my career have been driven by a strong intrinsic desire to help their patients, alleviate pain and suffering, cure disease, and restore patients to a state of wellness. It comes with the territory. Doctors are driven to master their craft and apply that skill in a way that delivers exceptional outcomes for patients. Physicians and other providers revel in the autonomy and high level of skill that accompanies being the "good doctor" (Berdud, Cabasés, and Nieto 2016). If doctors only went into medicine for the money, they would quickly realize there are much better ways to make a solid paycheck than to give up 10 to 15 years of their lives while incurring hundreds of thousands of dollars of debt, only to land at the bottom of the totem pole in a medical practice as the newbie.

Unfortunately, the extrinsic drivers of medical practice under the current fee-for-service medical system are too often misguided. Physicians and other health providers are expected to deliver transactional care—and lots of it. Providers are reimbursed for their time based on the resource-based relative value scale (RBRVS). Under the RBRVS system, providers are reimbursed for care they deliver based on visit complexity and/or timed aliquots. The more complex or lengthy the visit, the more the provider is reimbursed.

Healthcare has evolved into a big business in America in which the incentives have become increasingly geared toward high-tech, procedure-based service delivery where reimbursement is generous and splashy, bold marketing is common. Health systems and provider organizations have increasingly focused on the technology race to capture a larger market share. Unfortunately, as I will point out in this book, our technology addiction and misguided focus have driven us toward a system of inequity, extremely high cost, and diminishing outcomes.

As the United States recovers from its debilitated COVID state, it has become starkly evident that the current health system falls short of managing the individuals with the greatest illness burden and the social factors that impede health and longevity. One of the biggest challenges in improving this situation is that our current system incentivizes behavior that neither supports the health of a community nor helps people achieve wellness.

One of the biggest challenges in improving this situation is that our current system incentivizes behavior that neither supports the health of a community nor helps people achieve wellness.

THE ROARING INEFFICIENCIES OF AMERICAN MEDICAL CARE

I still remember where I was when I learned that a physician may receive greater reimbursement if a patient experiences an adverse event from the service they are receiving. I was in my internal medicine residency at the time and was working with a grizzled old physician who clearly had just about had it with the health system and with medicine in general.

"You know what the problem is here?" he said. "Too many people get their pockets lined by doing more procedures. Practices buy a new machine and apply it to everyone. If your favorite tool is a hammer, all the world looks like a nail." That was the first time I heard that expression, not realizing that he heard this from the behavioral scientists of the 1960s (Maslow 1962) or maybe that he was just a fan of Peter, Paul, and Mary.

"If you do a procedure and the patient has a complication, or it doesn't work, that just leads to a second procedure," he added.

I was the kind of trainee who always seemed to find a counterpoint—a true pain in the ass. "Wait a second," I responded. "There are consequences to subpar performance as a physician. What about reputation? What about reporting of outcomes? What about the innate desire to do a good job for those in your care? These things all seem to be in place to encourage better outcomes."

"I am not talking about bad docs with bad intentions," he replied. "Luckily, they are few and far between. I am talking about what drives doctors—or any operator, for that matter. I am talking about a system that is designed to encourage doctors to simply *do more*."

I don't think I knew exactly what he meant during that conversation, but I nodded and backed off politely so as not to focus his rising ire on me.

The US medical system is highly complex and inefficient. The United States spends more on healthcare than any other developed nation, with the highest percentage of gross domestic product devoted to healthcare expenditures (Organisation for Economic Co-operation and Development 2023). While the increased spending might be more tolerable if our outcomes were far superior, the US healthcare system consistently ranks poorly in key performance measures. According to the Commonwealth Fund (2021), the United States ranked *last* overall among 11 high-income countries in 71 performance measures in the following five categories:

- Care process
- Access to care
- Administrative efficiency
- Equity
- Healthcare outcomes

If the United States being last overall in the study's 71 performance measures was not bad enough, the researchers found that US healthcare also ranked dead last in each category except for care process. This book will share innovative solutions in all of the categories listed above, especially that last one.

RETHINKING REIMBURSEMENT

Reimbursement of medical care is similarly complex and inefficient. In our current system, a physician is typically eligible for reimbursement mainly for services delivered during a visit with a chronically ill patient, and the patient is pretty much responsible for what happens with their health during the time between their visits. What if we could somehow make the provider *eligible* for reimbursement for the patient's health-related outcomes? What if the patient and the provider are collectively accountable for health outcomes for not just one individual but all of their population? If we can change our focus, we will flip our perverse incentives on their heads.

What does all this mean to the American public? Have we left the health of our communities in the hands of corporate America? Or is there a way that providers can maintain clinical independence and create more effective incentives to focus on delivering wellness to their communities?

That is where population health and community wellness come in, and that is the subject of our next chapter.

REFERENCES

Berdud, M., J. M. Cabasés, and J. Nieto. 2016. "Incentives and Intrinsic Motivation in Healthcare." *Gaceta sanitaria* 30(6): 408–414. http://doi.org/10.1016/j.gaceta.2016.04.013.

Commonwealth Fund. 2021. "Mirror, Mirror 2021: Reflecting Poorly—Health Care in the US Compared to Other High-Income Countries." Published August 4. http://commonwealthfund.org/publications/fund-reports/2021/aug/mirror-mirror-2021-reflecting-poorly.

Maslow, A. H. 1962. *Toward a Psychology of Being.* New York: D Van Nostrand. http://doi.org/10.1037/10793-000.

Organisation for Economic Co-operation and Development (OECD). 2023. "Health Expenditure and Financing." Accessed May 8, 2023. https://stats.oecd.org/Index.aspx?ThemeTreeId=9.

Physicians Advocacy Institute. 2022. "PAI-Avalere Health Report on Trends in Physician Employment and Acquisitions of Medical Practices: 2019–2021." Updated April. http://physiciansadvocacyinstitute.org/PAI-Research/Physician-Employment-and-Practice-Acquisitions-Trends-2019-21.

Sinclair, U. 1934. *I, Candidate for Governor: And How I Got Licked.* New York: Farrar & Rinehart.

CHAPTER 2

Population Health: The Infinite Game

*Infinite-minded leaders don't ask their people to fixate on finite goals;
they ask their people to help them figure out a way to advance toward
a more infinite vision of the future that benefits everyone.*
Simon Sinek (2019)

As WITH EVERY encounter I have, I try to learn something interesting from my patients, and one particular shining star is Dr. Louis. At 79, Louis was a widowed, retired surgeon who still made an effort to wear a tie every day. He often smiled and told me stories about how he built his surgical practice by staying positive and "treating patients like my own family." I appreciated our conversations, and I think we all could learn something from Louis.

Early one Monday morning, Louis's daughter called my office to let me know her father had fallen and broken his hip while climbing the stairs at home. She was clearly upset. She worried about the statistics that showed poor outcomes for the elderly after hip fractures. She also knew her dad had diabetes and coronary artery disease, which required ongoing medical management. She worried whether he would make it through surgery and who would care for him afterwards. She worried how he would manage his chronic conditions in the setting of this new fracture.

After some medical optimization, Louis underwent successful surgery to repair his hip fracture. He was a real trouper when it came to his therapy. He was motivated to return to walking as quickly as possible, so he did every exercise the therapist gave him and more. I visited him in the rehab facility to check on his status. As I reviewed his chart, I saw he was on 11 medications. Most of them were different from what he was taking before his fall. Frustrated, he told me he was not able to follow the complex medication regimen that he was getting in the rehab facility.

As I sat with him, Louis confided that his biggest fear was to be a burden on his only daughter. "She is busy and has kids of her own," he said. "She doesn't need to worry about this old man."

Louis valued his independence more than any other aspect of his care. We spoke about his goals of care and how we would work together to achieve them. More than most, he understood the importance of keeping up with his health to maintain his independence. It would take months to get him back to his prior level of functioning and to help him feel in control of his medical care.

THE GRAYING OF AMERICA

The US population is aging. This inescapable fact of our existence affects all industries, including the world of healthcare, whether one is a patient, physician, payer, or politician.

In 2020, the US Census Bureau estimated that the population of those 65 years and older was 54.6 million people, which was nearly 17 percent of the population at that time (US Census Bureau 2020). Statisticians predict that by 2060 there will be 94.7 million people 65 years old or older, making up nearly one-quarter of the population (US Census Bureau 2018).

Equally sobering is that, according to the US Department of Health and Human Services (HHS), more than 10,000 people turn 65 each day (HHS 2022). In fact, in the not-too-distant future—2034 to be exact—the 65-and-over population is expected to outnumber children for the first time in US history (US Census Bureau 2018). As the population ages in some countries, more diapers are sold for adults than for children (Rich and Inoue 2021). The societal and financial implications are massive.

The graying of America affects not only the health of individuals but also the state of the American healthcare system in general. At the age of 65, much of the population is generally well. By the time one reaches 75, one might not be as functionally independent and may have a chronic health condition or two, but the odds are still favorable to remain functional with some assistance. At 85, one will likely have a chronic health condition (or several) that affects the ability to manage one's own care. Beyond 85, it becomes increasingly likely that someone will need assistance in their care, at the mercy of an industry where the payment models are strained and the workforce is stretched thin. The status of care of the aging American currently is not impressive, and the long-term-care industry is not adequately equipped to handle what is coming.

The effects on the healthcare industry are already being seen. Research from the consulting firm Gibbins Advisors in summer 2022 found that bankruptcies among large healthcare organizations are rising, and the trend is being led by long-term-care facilities. Researchers found that from the beginning of 2021 through June 2022, 30 large skilled-nursing and senior-care holding companies declared bankruptcy. This represents more than half of bankruptcies among large healthcare organizations during that period (Christ 2022).

This situation is potentially exacerbated by another key demographic that affects the aging population: dependents. US Census data shows that from 2010 to 2020, there was a 34 percent increase in the 65-and-older population. In fact, when comparing the non-working-age population (the dependent population) to those who are working, demographics show significant growth in the nonworking (dependent) sector (Rogers and Wilder, 2020). For the American health system to function properly as designed, we require younger, healthy, working-aged people to fuel the system. Not only does the working population provide physical care for the older generations, but they also pay taxes into a system that is designed to support the care of the Medicare patient.

According to projections from the Centers for Medicare & Medicaid Services (CMS), national health spending is expected to experience average annual growth of 5.4 percent between 2019 and 2028, reaching $6.2 trillion and increasing the share of the gross domestic product from 17.7 percent to 19.7 percent. At that point, one in five dollars paid in the United States will be spent on healthcare. According to these projections, healthcare spending will outpace GDP growth in each of those years. To make matters more challenging, Medicare spending exhibited an annual growth rate of 6.3 percent between 2000 and 2022, mostly because of costly new technology and growing enrollment from an aging population (KFF 2023).

This raises the question of where the money will come from to manage the health, well-being, chronic care, and long-term care of the aging population. With fewer producers in the market than people who are consuming goods and services, many things are going to change, and nearly every industry will be affected. It is easy to argue that the healthcare industry will feel those effects more than any other (Goodhart and Pradhan 2020).

CREATING POPULATIONS FROM PEOPLE

So far in this chapter, I have been addressing population demographics and financial considerations to illustrate the looming crisis in providing and paying for healthcare in a population with shifting demographics. To better understand how to manage this coming crisis, we will need to take a new path. The healthcare delivery system must adapt to create efficient pathways to provide the aging population with high-quality, equitable, and fiscally responsible outcomes that are far superior to those of the past.

This new paradigm of care should be based on values that are espoused by the population while delivering care congruent with individual goals. Interventions should be easy to access and consistent in their delivery. Managing the care of our communities requires that services emanate conveniently from all touchpoints between the population and the healthcare delivery system to reward wellness and foster the best possible outcomes.

Population health aggregates data on the distinct healthcare encounters of thousands of individuals who collectively make up a population. Population health takes a global look at wellness in a defined population to measure outputs. Those outputs include quality outcomes, disease-free survival, improved morbidity from disease, and resource stewardship (i.e., cost of care).

That's what I as a healthcare leader see as the value that the population health approach brings to the doctor–patient relationship. Let's explore how managing populations can lead to a stronger and more sustainable health system for all.

THE ELEMENTS OF POPULATION HEALTH MANAGEMENT

In a healthy population, we focus on preventive medicine, such as pap smears, mammograms, and vaccines. Solid medical practice focuses on evidence-based efforts to prevent disease. If that cannot be achieved, we strive to detect disease as early as possible, when it is most manageable and easiest to eradicate.

For those with chronic or severe illness, population health focuses on using a team-based approach for managing illness to prevent progression or exacerbation. Our job is to keep individuals as healthy as possible, out of the emergency department, and living life according to well-defined and shared goals.

In population health, we use a set of tools to drive the care of a group of individuals (see exhibit 2.1). We can categorize those tools as data observations and clinical interventions.

To start our journey, we collect data—big data. We look at demographics, healthcare access, delivery, who gets diseases, what

Exhibit 2.1. Key Elements of Population Health

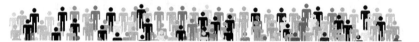

What Is Population Health ?

DATA OBSERVATIONS	CLINICAL INTERVENTIONS

BIG DEMOGRAPHICS

 Active collection of BIG DATA that provides an understanding of large populations, their patterns of use of resources, and their level of activity.

CARE MANAGEMENT

 Includes navigating the patient through the complex health system, ensuring proper follow-up, mitigating care gaps, and facilitating care transitions.

ROBUST ANALYTICS

 Looks for meaningful patterns in collected data and attempts to understand the current state, draw historical conclusions, and make accurate predictions.

WELLNESS PROGRAMS

 Promote health and wellness of population, including those with chronic conditions (healthy eating in diabetes, exercise in heart failure, etc.)

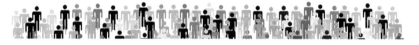

day of the week and time individuals are likely to present to the emergency room, medication use patterns, and more. Raw data contain huge amounts of information but lack insights needed for true understanding.

Robust analytics is needed to turn raw data into useful insights. Using intensive analytics, we aggregate large volumes of data to describe the overall health of a population while assessing where resources are needed most. Our analyses show us what is working well and what the areas of greatest concern are. We typically depict our aggregated data and insights in a dashboard using key performance indices for a given population.

Once we have our dashboard solidly in place, we can begin to identify the clinical resources that are needed to help move the needle on performance in specific areas. One typical clinical resource we use is care management. Care managers are nurses, pharmacists, physicians, or other providers who help a given individual navigate the highly complex health system. Care managers typically guide patients properly while understanding the patients' wishes and individual goals. Here they make sure patients keep their follow-up appointments, take their new medications as prescribed, and work to establish adequate home-based services to prevent further exacerbation. Care management is all about meeting individuals where they are, using shared decision-making, and helping to execute a plan that is consistent with the individual's goals. We will discuss this important component of care further in chapter 8.

Of course, no population health program would be complete without a focus on the wellness approach. Wellness programs include elements such as smoking-cessation classes, stress management sessions, and healthy-eating programs. It takes years of focus on wellness to decrease actual events such as heart attacks or strokes, but the return on investment is worthwhile. These programs are an important part of a comprehensive and balanced program for the community.

What is in this new paradigm of care?

- Accountability (from providers, payers, patients)
- Team-based care
- Care coordination
- Patient-focused goals of care
- Quality targets
- Equitable care delivery and outcomes
- Focus on efficiency and resource stewardship
- Wellness programs (e.g., smoking cessation, weight loss, exercise)
- Continuum management (home, acute care, post-acute care)

Unlike the incentives presented in chapter 1, population health programs are fueled by value-based payment models with insurers that deviate from the well-established production-line approach. *Value-based care* refers to a system of care that facilitates population health management—care based on value. Often, these terms are used interchangeably.

It is worth dispelling a common misconception regarding value-based care. Providing value-based care is not about cutting corners, being stingy, or withholding healthcare resources. Value-based care is about using evidence-driven treatment modalities and avoiding duplication and wasteful spending. Success is often driven by decreasing the use of acute care or the emergency department for conditions that should be managed in a primary care setting. Success also comes from listening to patients' wishes and helping them achieve their goals.

VALUE-BASED CARE AND ACCOUNTABLE CARE ORGANIZATIONS

In theory, value-based care is a relatively simple concept. Health insurers such as Medicare, Medicaid, or commercial insurers say, "Dr. Angelo, you practice in the Philadelphia community, and this is your group of patients that we have identified. Based on your population's illness burden and a few actuarial calculations, here is what we believe they should cost. We will pay you that amount. Manage these folks well."

Now the calculus is a bit different than it was in the legacy model of fee-for-service.

With that type of agreement—often called a value-based, risk-sharing, or population health agreement—I am expected to manage my patients (every one of them) using sound, evidence-based practice. I am also charged with being a good steward of the resources I have at my disposal. I am paid to keep a population well. Using evidence-guided practice resulting in fewer exacerbations and hospitalizations will decrease the cost of care.

This may sound a lot different from the healthcare system I described in chapter 1, in which the healthcare system makes more money if people get sicker. That kind of system will not survive the growing needs of an aging population. Finding a healthy way to bring those realities back from the brink of crisis requires that we become familiar with a term popularized by author and inspirational leader Simon Sinek: the infinite game.

Playing the Infinite Game

To understand the concept of the infinite game in healthcare, let us begin with a look at the flip side: the finite game. If I am a provider who is playing the finite game, I am focused on everything that happens during the 15 minutes I spend with a patient after walking into the room, because that's what I am getting paid for: delivery of a transaction. Do I properly diagnose a condition in that time frame? Do I deliver an exceptional patient experience? Do I have all the test results I need? Do I have all the equipment I need to manage the patient in that time? Do I communicate in a way that the patient can understand? Do I have the right knowledge to manage their medical problems? Does my documentation adequately reflect the content of our visit?

If answers to those questions are all yes, everything comes together, and I don't make the patient stay too long in the waiting room before seeing them, I will probably have a satisfied patient. In the finite game, I just checked all the right boxes. Mission accomplished, right?

Unfortunately, healthy patients and healthy perspectives do not always thrive in the finite world. Shifting our paradigm of care involves playing the infinite game. Patient health is not all about what happens in 15-minute aliquots every three months inside the examination room. It is more about what happens in the life of that patient—who continues to live on beyond those 15 minutes—and how I make sure that they can surmount any barriers they may encounter.

When physicians and other providers are providing care in a value-based, population health–focused environment, they are responsible not only for the 15 minutes of the visit but also for what happens in those 132,000 minutes between visits. If bad things happen to a patient during that intervening time, additional resources may be required to bring the patient back to health. Within this new paradigm of healthcare delivery, healthcare providers or provider organizations do not get a second installment of money if patients get sicker and must go to the emergency department or get admitted to the hospital.

When I am playing the infinite game, I have deeper questions to ask myself than I did in the finite game. How do I make sure someone's major social drivers of health needs are met? How do I make sure that a patient knows how to recognize the signs of exacerbation? How can they communicate if they have complications? Have we addressed the behavioral health aspects of care? How do we stay connected to catch disease exacerbation early and return the patient to health in a timely manner?

The solutions involved in value-based, population health–driven care are wide-ranging, and they involve healthcare systems, primary- and specialty-care providers, and commercial and governmental payers working together to

- partner with communities and community-based organizations to improve wellness and address inequitable care;
- create innovative systems that help patients navigate the complex and burdensome world of healthcare;
- use resources efficiently, even in systems with big financial challenges;

- thoughtfully apply technology to expand access to those who experience challenges to their basic daily needs (e.g., food, housing, and transportation); and
- change the reimbursement system, which simply rewards additional procedures, to a global payment system that encourages wellness and superior outcomes in a defined population.

This is the infinite game. It's not just about the 15 minutes. It's the life in between the visits that our efforts must involve.

Taking the Risk

Taking on the challenge of population health for providers involves taking on *risk*. What happens if my patients are sicker than antici-pated? What happens if my patients don't follow their plans of care? What if there is some other form of strain on the provider team, such as the COVID-19 pandemic? There is no doubt that delivering on the mission of population health involves a risk of failure. No innovative industry disruptor comes without risk. We as providers must understand that risk and work together to mitigate it.

There is no doubt that the risk of failure exists when it comes to delivering on the mission of population health. No innovative industry disruptor comes without risk.

Several organizational structures are available to help providers understand and succeed at the risk game. Some organizations will partially or even fully accept the risk on behalf of smaller practices in exchange for a larger portion of shared savings. Some payers, CMS included, will allow for a risk "glide path" that allows provider organizations to move slowly but steadily toward incrementally higher levels of risk. Strong analytics and clinical programs will come together to ensure that risk exposure is minimal.

To make a long story short, success in value-based care involves taking a risk.

Looking at the future of healthcare, provider organizations have arisen across the country to address the needs arising from value-based care and risk levels. One such entity is the accountable care organization (ACO). Chapter 4 will provide more detail about this type of organization. For now, it is important to understand that an ACO is a group of providers that collaborate and say, "We can do a better job at managing the health of our population, and we are willing to prove it."

What Does Accountable Care Look Like?

When I ask the question above, I am reminded of CMS Administrator Chiquita Brooks-LaSure's plenary address at the 2022 National Association of ACOs Conference, in which she spoke about accountable care and where our system is coming from versus where it needs to be:

> Our traditional payment systems incentivize providers to minimize time with each patient and focus on the quantity rather than the quality of care. For many patients, their healthcare experience is fragmented and confusing, resulting in a number of poor health outcomes. Our mission at CMS is not only to expand access to care but also to ensure that healthcare is meaningful to the people we serve. Accountable care is about putting people at the center of their care, holistically assessing their needs, and coordinating the care they need to thrive. (Brooks-LaSure 2022)

Doing a better job means that providers can focus on the quality of care delivery. Providers can also focus on the cost of care delivery while being good stewards of our resources. An ACO takes the lead on keeping the community in our charge healthy rather than making more money through the production of more widgets. Providers within an ACO deliver team-based care in an approach that delivers on issues such as high-quality, coordinated, and efficient care. ACO providers use tools such as care coordination, therapy and rehabilitation, integrated behavioral health, and medication management. ACOs also manage caregiver education and help with navigation and advanced-care planning for seriously ill patients who may no longer wish to go to the hospital.

To recognize where the value comes from in this new environment, we need to understand some additional foundational aspects of population health, because when you are involved in population health management, you are truly in an infinite game.

KEEPING PACE IN POPULATION HEALTH

Population health, as a method for creating and managing systems to transform our fragile and failing health system, has been emerging for decades. The definition of population health is a moving target as our methods evolve for managing people's health. The following description from the National Committee for Quality Assurance (NCQA) checks most of my boxes:

> Population health management is a model of care that addresses individuals' health needs at all points along the continuum of care, including in the community setting, through participation, engagement, and targeted interventions for a defined population. The goal of population health management is to maintain or improve the physical and psychosocial well-being of individuals and address health disparities through cost-effective and tailored health solutions. (NCQA 2021, 6)

The following are some of the foundational aspects of population health management:

- Keeping a keen focus on prevention and wellness, not just for individuals but for providers, the health system, and the entire community as well
- Recognizing that there are many contributing factors to health outcomes, including social, cultural, racial, financial, geographical, and educational issues, to name a few
- Identifying priorities and action steps through the use of robust population data and advanced analysis to identify priorities and target resources and actions
- Developing and involving partners throughout the community in delivering care and promoting prevention
- Creating innovative funding solutions with incentives for creating systems that support physicians in making the right choices, thus making it easier to do the right thing in population health and all patient encounters

The first item in the list above is especially important. A critical piece of population health and community wellness involves ensuring that the health system serving the community also stays healthy. Healthcare provider organizations that are "unwell" cannot lead the population to health and keep it healthy. They need to be sustainable and resilient to future challenges, such as the aging-population crisis presented earlier in this chapter. Later chapters will address this imperative through the concept of the Quintuple Aim, which supports the well-being of our frontline providers.

The second bullet point above—social factors that contribute to health outcomes—also deserves special emphasis. Social factors vary among members of different populations, and many of these factors have disproportionately negative effects on vulnerable and underrepresented minority members of our communities. The next chapter will focus on this major impediment to population health and community wellness: health equity.

REFERENCES

Brooks-LaSure, C. 2022. "Opening Plenary." National Association of Accountable Care Organizations Fall Conference. Video, 44:48. http://naacoslive.com/archive/6962.

Christ, G. 2022. "Nursing Homes, Senior Living Facilities Driving Healthcare Bankruptcies." *Modern Healthcare.* Published September 28. http://modernhealthcare.com/post-acute-care/nursing-homes-senior-living-facilities-driving-healthcare-bankruptcies.

Goodhart, C., and M. Pradhan. 2020. *The Great Demographic Reversal: Ageing Societies, Waning Inequality, and an Inflation Revival.* London: Palgrave MacMillan.

KFF. 2023. "The Facts About Medicare Spending." Published June. http://kff.org/interactive/the-facts-about-medicare-spending.

National Committee for Quality Assurance (NCQA). 2020. *Population Health Management: Meeting the Demand for Value-Based Care.* Published November 2. http://ncqa.org/wp-content/uploads/2021/02/20210202_PHM_White_Paper.pdf.

Rich, M., and M. Inoue. 2021. "A New Source of Fuel in an Aging Japan: Adult Incontinence." *New York Times.* Published November 15. http://nytimes.com/2021/11/15/world/asia/adult-diapers-japan.html.

Rogers, L., and K. Wilder. 2020. "Shift in Working Age Population Relative to Older and Younger Americans." Published June 25. https://www.census.gov/library/stories/2020/06/working-age-population-not-keeping-pace-with-growth-in-older-americans.html

Sinek, S. 2019. *The Infinite Game.* New York: Penguin Random House.

US Census Bureau. 2020. "Age and Sex Composition in the United States: 2020." Updated October 17, 2022. http://census.gov/data/tables/2020/demo/age-and-sex/2020-age-sex-composition.html.

———. 2018. "Older People Projected to Outnumber Children for First Time in US History." Updated October 8, 2021. https://www.census.gov/newsroom/press-releases/2018/cb18-41-population-projections.html.

US Department of Health and Human Services (HHS). 2022. "Aging." Updated April 27. http://hhs.gov/aging/index.html.

CHAPTER 3

Community Wellness: The Promise of More Equitable Outcomes

Of all of the forms of inequality, injustice in health is the most shocking and inhumane.
Martin Luther King, Jr.

LET'S REWIND FOR a moment to a fateful afternoon of an average day in a typically busy clinic early in my career as a physician. At the time, I was delivering primary care in a community office setting. I was covering for my office partner, who was out on maternity leave, and I saw a bunch of patients who were not known to me. In the midst of activity, I had a lovely encounter with a 40-something patient, Maria (not her real name). Maria was primarily Spanish speaking but understood English quite well. With my limited medical Spanish, we quickly determined together that we did not need an interpreter.

Maria was quick to smile, nod, and say, "Yes, doctor" to everything I said. As I quickly reviewed her record, I noticed she had a history of breast cancer, which had been treated several years ago. Aha. I knew exactly what to do. I quickly scoured the chart looking for evidence of BRCA testing (a blood test to determine whether she had DNA mutations that increase breast cancer risk). I did not find such testing, so I promptly brought this to her attention. I discussed the importance of breast cancer screening as well as genetic counseling in a woman of her demographic. She very politely nodded, seemingly acknowledging the importance of this intervention. As the encounter progressed, though, it became increasingly evident to me that Maria was telling me what she believed I wanted to hear.

At the end of the appointment, she nodded courteously and thanked me. I thanked her for our conversation and exited the room. I heard a rustling behind me, and I was somewhat surprised to see my office manager, Maureen, enter the room carrying a brown bag. She closed the door.

As often happens during a busy clinic session, I was running more than a half hour behind schedule at that time, so I dutifully moved on to my next patient and figured I would ask Maureen about the encounter later.

When I spoke to Maureen later that evening, I asked her about the brown bag and why she had the closed-door conversation with Maria. Maureen's response was jolting and altered my focus for the rest of my career: "You know she has no food in her house, right?"

No, I'd had no idea that Maria was suffering from food insecurity.

Perhaps if I had asked this nice woman the right questions, I would have found that out. Perhaps if I had used an interpreter for the encounter, Maria could have been connected to the right resources to help with her situation. The most fruitful part of the encounter for her was to leave the office with a bag of graham crackers and a few sample cans of Ensure.

I completely missed the opportunity to make an essential impact on Maria's health.

Later, I tried to call Maria to recover this missed opportunity. The next week was met with unanswered calls. I even sent a letter to her home as I was praying that she would contact me back. Unfortunately, for me and her, I was unable to reach her after several attempts. She never had any of the testing done as I ordered and never followed up with our office. Now I can only imagine the effect I could have had if I had understood Maria's true need and referred her to the right resources to help stabilize her home situation.

EQUITY IN POPULATION HEALTH

A sad and stark reality of society is that despite so many years of struggle and attention, there are members of our communities who remain marginalized for one or more reasons. Perhaps for some individuals this is because of their primary language, their country of origin, their sexual orientation, a disability, or the tone of their skin. Racial, gender, and ethnic inequality in American society represents an ongoing health crisis for us all.

Those of us who are charged with navigating our populations to health must keep this reality at the forefront of our understanding. Often, individuals in marginalized populations are the most vulnerable, with shorter life expectancy, lower-quality care, limited healthcare access, higher costs, and poorer overall health outcomes (National Academies of Sciences, Engineering, and Medicine 2017). It is crystal-clear that managing our most vulnerable populations is the right thing to do—socially, morally, and fiscally. As chapter 2 pointed out, our goal in population health and value-based care is to improve the health of our communities. Achieving health equity across all populations is a top priority in population health management.

Often, individuals in marginalized populations are the most vulnerable, with shorter life expectancy, lower-quality care, limited healthcare access, higher costs, and poorer overall health outcomes.

Health equity means many things to different people, so I want to provide a definition widely accepted by many organizations, including the Centers for Disease Control and Prevention (CDC). In a report whose goal was to build consensus around defining health equity, Robert Wood Johnson Foundation researchers define the term as follows:

Health equity means that everyone has a fair and just opportunity to be as healthy as possible. This requires removing obstacles to health such as poverty, discrimination, and their consequences, including powerlessness and lack of access to good jobs with fair pay, quality education and housing, safe environments, and health care. (Braveman et al. 2017, 1)

This passage defines the goal of health equity and the obstacles to receiving it. But what happens when health inequity is allowed to persist? According to the CDC (2022), "health inequities are reflected in differences in length of life; quality of life; rates of disease, disability, and death; severity of disease; and access to treatment." The CDC adds that overcoming health inequities will require a concerted effort that involves patients, providers, payers, and policymakers.

The obstacles to health and how they present themselves in the population explain why healthcare providers working with patients cannot alone achieve health equity. For example, there is only so much that we as health providers can do to mitigate root-cause issues such as poverty or discrimination; we also need to be part of a much larger population-health/community-wellness team. Given the importance of health equity, let's further dissect some of consequences of inequity on the health of the community.

EXAMINING THE OBSTACLES TO HEALTH

If we have learned anything in medicine in the past 50 years, it is that cancer outcomes are improved if diagnosed at an early stage, when disease is localized. Delayed presentation and diagnosis result in worse outcomes. The negative effect of diagnosis in later stages of malignancy is demonstrated in an intensive literature review published in *Obstetrics & Gynecology* in 2022. The authors discovered that not only are Black women nearly twice as likely as White women to die of uterine cancer, but also "the disparities pervade the entire spectrum of care, including risk factors, comorbidities, diagnosis, treatment, and outcomes" (Whetstone et al. 2022, 654). In its startling analysis the review found that only 54 percent of Black women presented to healthcare providers with localized disease, compared to 71 percent of White women.

The COVID-19 pandemic has further underscored the health disparities seen in communities of color, with worsened outcomes, higher incidence within the community, increased likelihood of needing hospitalization, and higher death rates (Khanijahani et al. 2021). The tragedy of excess mortality and morbidity related to social drivers of health should be enough impetus to convince one of the need for a focus on health equity.

It turns out that failing to address health equity also results in astronomical costs. Research released in summer 2022 by Deloitte warned that the cost of inequities related to race, socioeconomic status, and sex/gender in the US healthcare system could exceed $1 trillion in annual spending by 2040 if we don't start doing something about them today. At the time of the report, the annual cost of these inequities was $320 billion (Davis et al. 2022). The report's authors state that the way to avoid this unsustainable level of spending while improving healthcare outcomes is for leaders and organizations to immediately begin "addressing the drivers of health, removing biases and inefficiencies in care, and enabling data and technology to help monitor, diagnose, and deliver care."

These drivers of health are known widely as "social determinants of health," though the naming convention for the social factors that affect health outcomes is not fully agreed upon. While many refer to these factors as social determinants of health, others take a different view—that social factors do not necessarily determine one's path—so they refer to them as social *drivers* of health. I, along with many in the population health community, believe that "social drivers of health" is a more accurate term.

THE IMPORTANCE OF ADDRESSING SOCIAL FACTORS IMPACTING HEALTH

Many of the gaps in health equity in our society and patient populations are related more to social factors than to genetics. Social drivers of health are defined by the World Health Organization (WHO) as "conditions in which people are born, grow, work, live, and age, and the wider set of forces and systems shaping the conditions of daily life. These forces and systems include economic policies and systems, development agendas, social norms, social policies, and political systems" (WHO 2022, 1).

There are innumerable examples of the social drivers of health in various communities. For instance, some of us are fortunate enough to reside in areas with abundant markets and fresh food availability so that we can maintain a diet of healthful options. Meanwhile, others may reside in what is known as a "food desert," where they have very limited access to supermarkets with healthy, high-quality food options and the only affordable options in that community are fast food. Likewise, in some of those same communities, burning the calories and fat from consuming those foods is a challenge. Safety may be such a grave issue in some neighborhoods that walking or jogging to maintain a level of fitness is more perilous than just sitting at home.

Some of the most important drivers are related to people's health in subtle or unexpected ways. If you didn't know anything about social drivers of health and were asked to name what you thought was the top one, transportation would probably not be your first choice. However, a lack of transportation is one of the biggest and most impactful barriers to health that individuals in America can encounter. People who lack transportation may lack social connections, access to healthy food, and access to healthcare. Poor mobility often results in inability to get into chronic disease management programs or access their primary care physicians. Similarly, if you can't get to the pharmacy to pick up your prescription, medication adherence is out of the question.

Of the many social drivers of health, most concern a few broad areas: access to high-quality care, access to high-quality education, economic resources, and the safety of communities in which people live. Typically, social drivers of health do not exist in a vacuum, and individuals may experience multiple dimensions of them. Exhibit 3.1 below shows the five domains of social drivers of health that are the areas targeted for improvement efforts by the US Department of Health and Human Services (HHS) Healthy People 2030 initiative (HHS 2020).

Exhibit 3.1. Social Drivers of Health

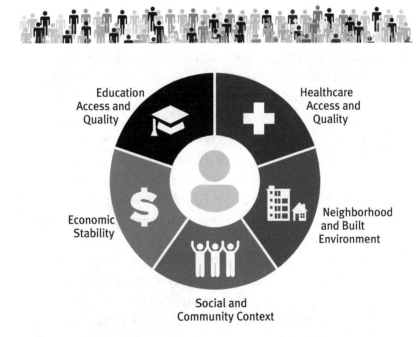

Source: Adapted with permission from HHS (2020).

When people think of social drivers of health, poverty usually comes to mind, but as exhibit 3.1 shows, many factors are involved in social drivers of health:

- *Economic stability.* People with steady employment are more likely to be healthy and less likely to live in poverty. They are also more likely to have health insurance, which can pay for preventive health services. But many people have difficulty finding and holding on to well-paying jobs for various reasons. Health can be one of them—people with disabilities and chronic conditions are often limited in the kind of work they can do.

- *Education access and quality.* Getting a job that pays a living wage is largely determined by access to high-quality education. Individuals who grow up in areas with underfunded schools that perform poorly start life at a great disadvantage. These individuals are also less likely to have families who can afford to support them in gainful higher education.

- *Healthcare access and quality.* More than 10 percent of people in the United States lack health insurance, which means that they don't have access to a primary care provider (PCP)—the foundation of healthcare access. Lack of access to medical care results in inadequate utilization of preventive services and delays in treatment until health status is at a critical stage. Sometimes people live too far away from high-quality healthcare providers because they are shuttered in their communities. Individuals with limited or inappropriate access to comprehensive primary care will often end up utilizing resources such as the emergency department (ED) for acute care. As a site of service, the ED is expensive and simply not focused on chronic condition management.

- *Neighborhood and built environment.* Many environments in neighborhoods around the United States are not conducive to promoting the health and safety of their residents. Often, these neighborhoods are populated by people with low incomes and/or by racial and ethnic minorities. People in these neighborhoods are often subjected to violence, unsafe air and water, and many other health and safety hazards.

- *Social and community context.* People in affluent neighborhoods generally have a wide range of social and community support available to them where they live and work. This is not usually the case in low-income neighborhoods, where community and social-support organizations are lacking. If they are in crisis—for example, being unable to afford food, clothing, transportation, and healthcare—they often have few options for getting help (HHS 2020).

FURTHER SOCIAL DRIVERS OF HEALTH

The COVID-19 pandemic laid bare many of the inequities in testing and treatment, vaccination, education, care access, quality, and health outcomes experienced by people from underrepresented minority groups in our populations. Primary care access has been and remains a problem in these communities.

Since early April 2020, when CMS sent a letter to all Medicare organizations approving reimbursement for the expansion of "virtual care" to reduce the risk of spreading the coronavirus, the use of telehealth rapidly expanded. This revolution has been positive for population health in many ways, especially for meeting people where they want to receive their care and helping alleviate some of the effects of transportation issues on PCP access.

For some people, that is.

Telehealth has been generally welcomed with open arms by providers and patients alike. Before the COVID-19 pandemic, I had seen zero telehealth patients. Now 10 to 20 percent of encounters during a typical clinic session for me may be telehealth encounters. When we were transitioning to our telehealth options, I assumed that the biggest roadblock we would run into would be low technical literacy. It wasn't. The greatest impediment was a lack of connectivity. No Wi-Fi. No broadband. And no way to pay for it.

Poverty is behind many of the social drivers I mentioned earlier, including broadband access, lack of health insurance, food insecurity, housing insecurity, lack of education, and limited access to transportation. These economic hardships often result in individuals relying on poorly paying jobs or inadequate social programs to mitigate their challenges. Their resultant effects increase chronic stress and even isolation, thus worsening the predicament for many in the community.

ADDRESSING THE CONTINUUM OF CARE

As a practicing hospice and palliative care physician and a leader in value-based care, I continue to see health inequities in my practice and in healthcare delivery in general. Overcoming the negative social drivers of health starts with an understanding of the continuum of care—how we follow patients through their journey within the health system. We will dive deeply into the continuum of care in chapter 8, but this is a good point to address the disparities that impede it.

Exhibit 3.2 is a graphic representation of the patient journey and highlights disparities in care along that journey. We start off considering individuals who reside within the community. These folks may be well overall or may have some health condition. The first and typically most appropriate access point to the healthcare continuum is through a PCP.

Exhibit 3.2. Disparities in the Continuum of Care

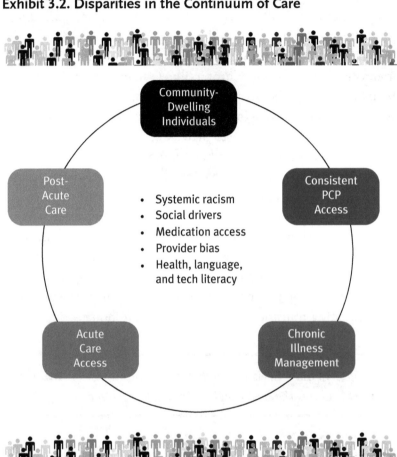

PCPs can assess, diagnose, and typically treat many chronic illnesses. They may refer complex patients to a specialty care physician for an opinion or a procedure. Ultimately, the PCP is the owner of the relationship with the patient and has the best insight into whole-person care. The best PCPs will use specialty care where appropriate and receive patients back from specialists in a co-management or collaborative model.

A surprising portion—nearly 60 percent—of adults suffer from at least one chronic illness (Buttorff, Ruder, and Bauman 2017). Typically, a chronic illness is defined as one that requires medical intervention, lasts more than a year, and may affect physical or emotional well-being. Chronic-illness management requires a thoughtful, comprehensive, team-based approach. PCPs are often the most adept at managing chronic illness, and they require the resources of team-based care to manage serious illness.

Value-based-care platforms help support these teams of nurses, social workers, pharmacists, behavioral health providers, dieticians, and more. A prime example of this is when a patient requires the skill of a dedicated care manager for their chronic disease navigation. These resources are integral to an accountable care organization. A skilled care manager will assist in navigating patients through the complex health system, ensuring proper follow-up, educating patients and caregivers, mitigating gaps that are discovered in care, and facilitating transitions from the hospital to home.

Ultimately, the PCP is the owner of the relationship with the patient and has the best insight into whole-person care.

People with chronic illnesses such as heart failure, lung disease, or diseases of the liver and kidneys may experience acute complications that may result in the need for acute care utilization. Acute care utilization often involves accessing the ED and/or an acute care hospitalization. Nowadays, the acute care setting is mainly used for the purpose of identifying and stabilizing the acute issue, such as treating an infection or administering some intervention that cannot be delivered in another setting. Typically, the acute care setting is the shortest stop along the care continuum.

If an individual is stabilized in an acute care environment, that patient will be discharged to post-acute care. Post-acute settings most frequently include management in the home, with or without professional support. This is the period when patients recover from their illnesses and return to their pre-hospitalization level of function if possible. If an individual's needs exceed the capacity of the patient and their family to safely navigate the home, an inpatient facility may be used for a short time to bridge their eventual return to the home.

CONTINUUM INEQUITIES

In addition to strong primary care, effective population health models require that members of a community have consistent access to their providers for preventive services and chronic care management. Unfortunately, individuals in underrepresented, marginalized populations often have substandard access to PCPs and specialty care physicians. If these individuals run into problems, they have no choice—they must go to the ED. Because of a lack of appropriate disease screening and attention to wellness, these folks are typically diagnosed with later-stage illness and may face fewer viable treatment options to return them to a state of wellness.

In the palliative care arena in which I practice, Black patients are particularly underserved. In 2021, the Project Equity workgroup of the Center to Advance Palliative Care (CAPC) conducted a comprehensive review of the peer-reviewed literature to learn more about healthcare and quality-of-life issues for Black individuals who live with serious illnesses and their families. Among their findings were that Black people living with serious illness experienced

- poorer-quality pain management from their providers,
- worse non-pain symptom management than White patients,
- an increased need for high-acuity care,
- higher medical costs during the course of their illness,
- fewer advanced-care planning discussions or documents (e.g., a living will or advanced directive) compared to White patients,

- mistrust of the healthcare system, and
- cultural factors that influence healthcare decision-making and are at odds with their health providers (CAPC 2021).

Solving inequities in the continuum of care will require wide-ranging determination on the part of people and organizations in every community. The Institute for Healthcare Improvement has been developing a consensus in the healthcare quality improvement community around what it calls the Triple Aim of better health outcomes, improved patient experience, and lower costs. More recently, thought leaders have added key areas of provider well-being and equity to these goals, as shown in exhibit 3.3.

Healthcare through the lens of the Quintuple Aim is beneficial for individuals and communities. The American health system will not succeed in its journey of transformation without clear focus on each of these areas. This is the path of healing for a health system

Exhibit 3.3. The Quintuple Aim

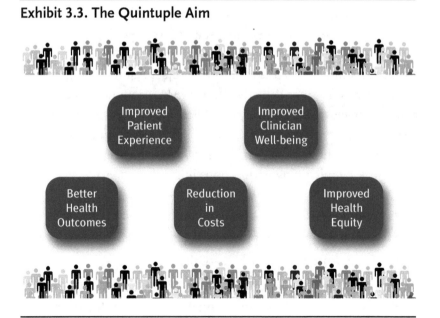

Source: Coleman et al. (2016).

that is bruised by a fee-for-service mentality; addicted to the latest, greatest technology; and hemorrhaging money as the life expectancy of Americans decreases.

To achieve population health and community wellness, we need to close gaps in the continuum of care, many of which I explained earlier in this chapter. Accountable care organizations are built on a platform of comprehensive population health management and equity in care. The next chapter will explore how accountable care organizations can help us move on from an ailing system to create a new paradigm of care delivery with a focus on quality, outcomes, and cost for all populations.

REFERENCES

Braveman, P., E. Arkin, T. Orleans, D. Proctor, and A. Plough. 2017. *What Is Health Equity? And What Difference Does a Definition Make?* Robert Wood Johnson Foundation. Published May 17. https://rwjf.org/content/dam/farm/reports/reports/2017/rwjf437343.

Buttorff, C., T. Ruder, and M. Bauman. 2017. *Multiple Chronic Conditions in the United States.* RAND Corporation. http://rand.org/pubs/tools/TL221.html.

Center to Advance Palliative Care. 2021. "Health Care for Black Patients with Serious Illness: A Literature Review." Updated August. http://capc.org/health-care-for-black-patients-with-serious-illness-a-literature-review.

Centers for Disease Control and Prevention (CDC). 2022. "Health Equity for People with Disabilities." Updated September 23. http://cdc.gov/ncbddd/humandevelopment/health-equity.html.

Coleman, K., E. Wagner, J. Schaefer, R. Reid, and L. LeRoy. 2016. *Redefining Primary Care for the 21st Century.* Agency for Healthcare Research and Quality. AHRQ Publication 16(17)-0022-EF. http://ahrq.gov/sites/default/files/wysiwyg/professionals/systems/primary-care/workforce-financing/white_paper.pdf.

Davis, A., N. Batra, A. Dhar, J. Bhatt, W. Gerhardt, and B. Rush. 2022. "US Health Care Can't Afford Health Inequities." *Deloitte Insights*. Published June 22. https://www2.deloitte.com/us/en/insights/industry/health-care/economic-cost-of-health-disparities.html

Khanijahani, A., S. Iezadi, K. Gholipour, S. Azami-Aghdash, and D. Naghibi. 2021. "A Systematic Review of Racial/Ethnic and Socioeconomic Disparities in COVID-19." *International Journal for Equity in Health* 20(1): 1–30. http://equityhealthj.biomedcentral.com/articles/10.1186/s12939-021-01582-4.

National Academies of Sciences, Engineering, and Medicine. 2017. "The State of Health Disparities in the United States." In *Communities in Action: Pathways to Health Equity*, edited by A. Baciu, Y. Negussie, and A. Geller. Washington, DC: National Academies Press. http://ncbi.nlm.nih.gov/books/NBK425844.

US Department of Health and Human Services (HHS). 2020. "Social Determinants of Health." Healthy People 2030. Accessed April 9, 2023. http://health.gov/healthypeople/objectives-and-data/social-determinants-health.

Whetstone, S., W. Burke, S. S. Sheth, R. Brooks, A. Cavens, K. Huber-Keener, D. M. Scott, B. Worly, and D. Chelmow. 2022. "Health Disparities in Uterine Cancer: Report from the Uterine Cancer Evidence Review Conference." *Obstetrics & Gynecology* 139(4): 645–59. https://doi.org/10.1097/AOG.0000000000004710.

World Health Organization (WHO). 2022. "Social Determinants of Health." Accessed April 9, 2023. https://www.who.int/health-topics/social-determinants-of-health.

CHAPTER 4

Accountable Care Organizations

Healthy citizens are the greatest asset any country can have.
Winston Churchill

A RECENT CALL with a former colleague of mine, Tony, reminded me of the importance of meeting patients where they want to be. Tony was exasperated as he called me to talk about his concerns for the well-being of his significant other, Kim.

Kim is a highly educated woman and a seasoned healthcare worker who knows the signs to watch for exacerbation of her chronic illness. When she began to notice signs of a problem, she called her hematologist. Unfortunately, her hematologist was out of the country. The covering physician had little knowledge of her case and quickly told Kim to go to the nearest hospital for evaluation.

Kim knew that the nearest hospital was one where her specialists were not affiliated, but she was frightened, and she knew the nearest hospital was a particularly well-known and highly regarded institution. So she did as she was told, and Tony drove Kim over to the nearest emergency department (ED).

The ED was busy and had little information about her case. The staff at the facility were very nice to her, though they informed her that they would not be able to arrange for home services and admitted her to the hospital.

Once in the acute-care setting, Kim quickly grew confused and frustrated, and she felt out of control. She did not know her physicians, and no one contacted her regular hematologist to ask her what her prior treatment course had been. She heard conflicting opinions about her care and was unclear about who was in charge of her case.

As Tony told me of Kim's difficulties, I did my best to actively listen while supporting him. "I can only imagine how difficult it has been," I told him in my best palliative-care-provider tone.

Tony responded, "Actually, I don't think you can."

He explained further: "Every night they wake her up at several points to make sure she is feeling OK. Blood draws happen at 6 a.m. For days, the staff has informed her that she cannot eat because she is going to have a procedure at 10. Then it doesn't happen at 10, and it doesn't happen at 12, and eventually they say it is going to be the next day. By then she has skipped two meals and is told, 'We're really sorry, but it's too late to order food now. We should be able to get you a sandwich for dinner.'

"She is visited by residents, interns, nurses, and students more than 15 times per day. Different specialists discuss their divergent thoughts and approaches with her while she is on pain medications, sometimes before the sun comes up. You cannot imagine how wildly the plan changes from day to day. She really can't keep up with these conversations.

"All she wants to do is be discharged. She has been told it will happen multiple mornings now with no one following up to tell her if it is a 'go' or not. As a rule, nothing happens on the weekend. Nothing. I just don't see a lot of healing going on there."

Kim is a patient who is not where she wants to be.

So much of population health is about meeting patients along their healthcare journey where they want to be during their healthcare journey. This is true in a metaphorical sense as we walk with patients toward a desired health goal, and it is also true literally when we provide care at the location of the patient's choosing. What is important to someone as a patient should be important to us as providers, and this is a big issue.

PICKING THE RIGHT SITE OF SERVICE

If someone's goal as a patient of the health system is to stay home to receive care even though they may have a chronic illness with intermittent exacerbations, we in the health system should try our best to keep that individual well-managed at home. We should not try to have individuals meet us where we are, which often means that they have to go to the hospital.

The physician in me recognizes the importance of hospital-based, acute care delivery. I have worked with many health systems in my career, and they are often adept at delivering the kind of care they know how to deliver best: inpatient care. Hospital inpatient-care teams are often robust and consist of physicians, nurses, dieticians, pharmacists, therapists, social workers, and a host of other professionals. Hospitals leverage their resources to give patients the care they need to get through acute illness in the finite period. Hospitals are especially skillful at picking up a patient in an exacerbated state, dusting them off, and getting them back out the door and on their way to recovery. Acute care delivery is an essential segment of our health system, but alone it does not translate into long-term health outcomes.

Acute care delivery is an essential segment of our health system, but alone it does not translate into long-term health outcomes.

ACCOUNTABLE CARE ORGANIZATIONS DEFINED

Because acute care delivery (that is, hospital care) does not result in long-term positive health outcomes on its own, something else is needed to focus on longitudinal care, give proper attention to preventive care and chronic condition management, and provide long-term patient engagement. Accountable care organizations (ACOs) bring that skill set to patient care.

In chapter 1, we examined the incentives that drive behavior in the healthcare delivery system. Then in chapter 2, we began to explore the concept of population health and the ACO as a model for delivering high-quality care with a focus on outcomes. An ACO is defined as an aggregator of physicians and other providers who strive to improve the health and lives of their population through collaboration and who focus on quality care delivery and resource stewardship. This chapter will explore accountable care from its origins to where we are today.

THE HISTORY OF ACCOUNTABLE CARE

An ACO is a group of providers who work collaboratively to improve cost and quality of care delivery for a defined population, rewarding both efficiency and wellness. ACOs can be organized in different ways: by geographic area, by criteria set by governmental and commercial payer programs, by the particular aims of the collaborating providers, by a specific patient population's needs (e.g., kidney failure), or some combination of these. An ACO's focus typically starts with primary care for wellness and disease management and prevention. ACOs also focus on comprehensive care coordination for patients with chronic conditions who need complex and costly medical or surgical interventions.

The original idea behind ACOs was to drive the US healthcare system away from the fee-for-service model, which I introduced in chapter 1, and toward value-based care. In other words, the movement was toward value rather than volume, with the *value* in value-based care defined as creating better health outcomes for people.

An ACO is a group of providers who work collaboratively to improve cost and quality of care delivery for a defined population, rewarding both efficiency and wellness.

In 2005, the Centers for Medicare and Medicaid Services (CMS) began creating what we now call ACOs with its Medicare Physician Group Practice Demonstration, which was ended in 2010. As with ACOs, risk for treating populations was moved toward provider groups, but the model still relied on traditional fee-for-service billing. While cost of care and quality success was achieved by some of the provider groups in the demonstration project, results were generally mixed (Tu et al. 2015).

The formal recognition of ACOs commenced with the Patient Protection and Affordable Care Act of 2010 (ACA). The promotion of ACOs was one of the top reforms of the ACA, which was developed to improve the US healthcare system by providing incentives for enhancing quality, improving beneficiary outcomes, and increasing value.

In January 2012, Medicare introduced its Pioneer ACO Program, followed that April by the launch of the Medicare Shared Savings Program. A foundational concept of these programs and those that came after has been shared risk and reward for performance. Since then, the concept has been moving gradually toward ACOs taking on more risk.

It is important to note here that value-based care is considered an area of healthcare legislation that garners bipartisan support in Washington. Both Republican and Democratic leaders have recognized the importance of high-quality and efficient care delivery. A prime example of this bipartisanship is a letter sent in late 2022 and signed by 28 Democrat and 15 Republican House members urging Congress to include Section 4 of the *Value in Health Care Act* (H.R. 4587) in an end-of-year legislative package. This push was intended to extend the 5 percent Alternative Payment Model (APM) incentive payments under the Medicare Access and CHIP Reauthorization Act and to allow CMS to adjust qualifying criteria. The letter states: "We ask that you continue paving the path toward value-based care that Congress and the Centers for Medicare and Medicaid Services (CMS) have been striving for by ensuring more patients are able to access integrated care at lower costs by providers in APMs" (Bailey 2022).

RISKY BUSINESS

Up to this point, we have referenced the concept of *risk*, as in providers taking on risk or sharing risk. We touched on it in chapter 2 as well. Let's take a moment here to review this important concept in some depth.

Exhibit 4.1 shows how the design of accountable care can be depicted through the risk continuum. As providers move from historical fee-for-service models of payment, they move toward the next stop along the continuum, where organizations still receive fee-for-service payments but may receive a bonus for completing some specified quality activities. These activities include elements such as infection reduction or percentage completion of various screening activities for a population.

Next on the risk glidepath is a provider organization that receives some additional reimbursement if certain financial thresholds are

Exhibit 4.1. Risk Continuum

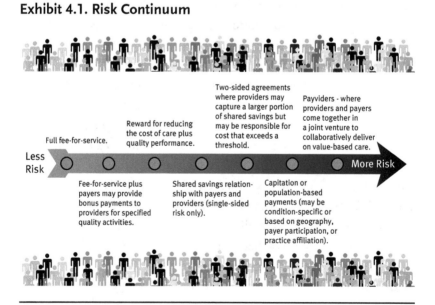

reached. These thresholds could be based on market trends or historical cost trends and then adjusted based on the illness burden for a population. Patients with a higher burden of accurately documented illness are expected to cost more.

Shared-savings arrangements can include single-sided risk (also known as "upside-only") or two-sided risk. In single-sided risk, a provider organization is held accountable for the total cost of care and can receive additional funding if the total cost is less than predicted. In a two-sided risk agreement, provider organizations can receive shared savings if targets are achieved, or they may be held accountable (downside risk) if the cost of care is significantly higher than predicted (see exhibit 4.2).

Moving further along the spectrum, we have full-risk programs. These programs are based on population-based payments or capitation. Full risk means that an organization is reimbursed for the illness profile of its population, and it is expected to manage its population with the resources provided. It is appropriate that additional risk incursion offers the opportunity for additional funding for providers.

Finally, we come to the payvider relationship, in which a provider organization and a payer come together in a collaborative business structure to manage a population. Generally, these partnerships are created to advance the delivery of services to a population with a focus on evidence-based practice, exceptional patient experience, and superior outcomes. These joint ventures can take any number of shapes and often involve rewards for population-focused care. I will present more information about the payvider arrangement in chapter 5.

ACCOUNTABLE CARE TODAY AND TOMORROW

According to the National Association of ACOs, in January 2023 there were 456 Medicare Shared Savings Program ACOs and 132 ACO Reach entities serving more than 13 million beneficiaries across

Exhibit 4.2. Shared Savings Scenarios

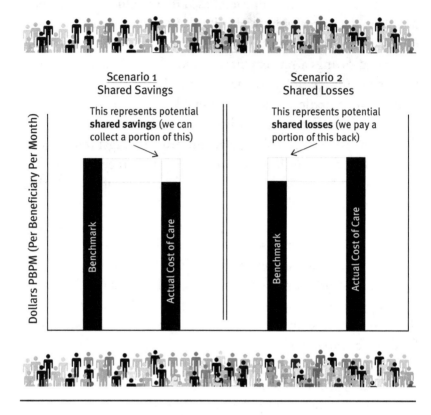

the country. That number has increased significantly since inception. In fact, CMS has set a goal for all Medicare fee-for-service beneficiaries to be in a "care relationship with accountability for quality and total cost of care by 2030" (CMS 2021).

Individuals who live in the population that benefits from this new model of healthcare delivery are called *beneficiaries* because they are receiving benefits often covered by governmental payers. We also often refer to these individuals as beneficiaries of the ACO. The benefits given through ACO participation may include some or all of the following:

- Coordinated services with careful navigation through the complex healthcare delivery system

- Preventive care
- Dedicated medication therapy management
- Integrated behavioral health
- Wellness coaching
- Identification and mitigation of social factors affecting health
- Collaborative medical care through close provider communication
- Superior access to care
- A focus on quality outcomes
- Transparency of all aspects of the care continuum

ACOs are driven by data. Good data make for good decisions. An ACO's data are collected on various populations to support positive outcomes and drive down excessive costs. For instance, if we find that a population has poor outcomes in breast cancer or low levels of breast cancer screenings, an ACO will embark on a campaign to encourage the population to receive more timely mammograms for early breast cancer detection. Similarly, if utilization patterns show that the people in a given geographical area are prone to using the ED for primary care, additional access to primary care physicians in that region may help. Chapter 6 will dive deeper into how we use data in value-based care.

Unfortunately, many patients are not even aware that they are beneficiaries of an ACO. Typically, patients are attributed to the organization through their primary physician, who has enrolled in such an agreement.

The lack of patient engagement in the value-based care model has been one of the major criticisms of ACOs over the years. ACOs and population health–focused organizations have done an inadequate job of informing patients of the benefits of participation in a value-based arrangement.

THE IMPORTANCE OF CARE RETENTION

When we talk about managing our population in an ACO model, it is important that we have visibility of what is happening at all stages of the continuum of care. In addition to having an awareness of a patient's living circumstances, all providers who are involved in a case must communicate seamlessly and leverage care that will contribute to that patient's long-term wellness. One way we address the need to see and manage our patients throughout the continuum is through care retention to our network.

Care retention refers to keeping a patient's care within a narrow network of providers. Those providers are often vetted for high quality and safety outcomes and a strong ability to deliver a good patient experience and to manage patients while paying attention to resource utilization. Many ACOs have rigorous network development teams to explore which providers are delivering exceptional outcomes and which ones may need some education or assistance with processes to improve performance.

One particular expert in this area is Mark Whalen, enterprise chief strategy officer from Jefferson Health, which is part of the large academic Thomas Jefferson University system in the greater Philadelphia region. When I discussed the topic of care retention with Mark, he emphasized the value of provider network development:

> Providers have an opportunity to best manage a population if the members of that population are seen within a clinically integrated group of providers. Activities such as acute-care hospitalizations or tests and procedures that happen outside the network can lack coordination. It is harder to manage a population that is not within our reach. We have extensively developed our network of providers over the years to focus on meaningful, high-quality outcomes and resource stewardship.

MODELS OF SUCCESS IN ACCOUNTABLE CARE

On its Innovation Models website, CMS provides case studies of ACOs throughout the United States that have developed innovative value-based programs that have improved beneficiary outcomes and resulted in reduced costs to the healthcare system (CMS 2023). I have chosen a few of the best practices that address several of the challenges I have covered so far. The following are three examples that demonstrate an extra layer of care given to beneficiaries:

1. **Preventing avoidable admissions.** Reliance Healthcare, an ACO in southwest Michigan, developed an ED care-coordination program intended to improve outcomes for people who present to different EDs throughout the region. The focus of the program is prevention of avoidable inpatient admissions by delivering care to beneficiaries in a lower-cost setting. The ED care-coordination program combines a centralized team of nurses that reviews cases with an information technology platform that enables communication between the ACO and ED personnel. When a beneficiary of the ACO presents at any of the EDs in the state, the care coordination team is alerted; after determining whether the ED is part of its network, the team goes to work first evaluating the case and then initiating the care-coordination process. This program not only reduces costs but also helps population health and community wellness efforts by improving provider-to-provider communication, arranging for follow-up care, and identifying beneficiaries who may need social services.

2. **Closing care gaps by meeting people where they want to be.** Keystone ACO, which primarily serves rural

areas in Pennsylvania, is a good example of combining population health and community wellness to create a program that serves unmet healthcare and social needs. Its Health Navigator Program employs a three-stage process. First, beneficiaries are flagged by predictive analytics or are referred to the program internally by primary care providers and other care team members. Then a community health assistant is assigned to the beneficiary and develops information on the beneficiary from information technology systems and from a nurse case manager. The community health assistant also conducts a home visit with the beneficiary to gather further information. At the third stage of the process, the nurse case manager and community health assistant jointly triage the patient to determine and address both clinical and nonclinical needs, connecting the beneficiary with appropriate clinical care and available community services. The program has received widespread positive feedback from both clinicians and beneficiaries and has created a novel hybrid career path involving population health and community wellness—the community health assistant.

3. **Coordinating care for high-cost/high-utilization beneficiaries.** In 2016, OneCare Vermont created a community care coordination program for beneficiaries deemed to be high risk on the basis of their previous healthcare use. The program uses predictive modeling to stratify the population into one of four categories using EHR information from the population. The categories range from 1, in which beneficiaries are a low illness burden (meaning that they are healthy and have limited or unavoidable utilization of the healthcare system) to 4, in which beneficiaries experience a high illness burden (meaning that they have complex needs or a

heavy burden of chronic conditions). These indicators
of needs can include a patient's number of medications,
frequency of ED admissions, non-adherence to treatment,
communication barriers, and stable housing access. Once
a beneficiary is enrolled, a care coordinator conducts
a detailed assessment to identify needs, care gaps, and
priorities for a care plan to determine which roles are
needed in the beneficiary's care team. Care teams often
include a care coordinator, social workers, primary care
physicians, case managers, mental health counselors, and
nutritionists. Enrollment in the program was lower than
expected for the first few years but jumped significantly,
from 504 beneficiaries in 2018 to more than 3,100 in 2020.
Results of the program included a 33 percent drop in
ED use for Medicare enrollees and a 13 percent drop for
Medicaid enrollees.

The central role of ACOs is to support primary care physicians in
caring for beneficiaries by keeping information on their health and
care updated while helping individuals make smarter decisions about
managing their health. This works only when the system makes the
individual, rather than the system itself, the focus of the healthcare
delivery system. This is how we address the most vulnerable members—both clinically and socially—of our populations, bridging
barriers and delivering care that is at once innovative and rooted in
evidence-guided medical practice.

As you will see in the rest of this book, creating a new paradigm
of care is not easy and does not happen without disruption to the
status quo. ACOs are one example of reimagining organizations
to meet the aims of value-based care. Another example is breaking
down the barriers and silos that have long existed among payers and
providers. That is the subject of the next chapter.

REFERENCES

Bailey, V. 2022. "Bipartisan Letter Requests Extended Value-Based Payment Incentives." *Revcycle Intelligence*. Published November 4. http://revcycleintelligence.com/news/bipartisan-letter-requests-extended-value-based-payment-incentives.

Centers for Medicare and Medicaid Services (CMS). 2023. "Accountable Care Organizations (ACOs): General Information/Case Studies." Updated April 13. http://innovation.cms.gov/innovation-models/aco.

—————. 2021. "Innovation Center Strategy Refresh." Published October 20. https://innovation.cms.gov/strategic-direction-whitepaper.

Tu, T., D. Muhlestein, S. L. Kocot, and R. White. 2015. *The Impact of Accountable Care: Origins and Future of Accountable Care Organizations*. Brookings Institution. Published May. http://brookings.edu/wp-content/uploads/2016/06/impact-of-accountable-careorigins-052015.pdf.

CHAPTER 5

Payviders: Symbiosis to Drive Value-Based Care

I think healthcare is more about love than about most other things. If [love] isn't at the core of these two human beings who have agreed to be in a relationship where one is trying to help relieve the suffering of another . . . you can't get to the right answer here.
Donald Berwick, former administrator of the Centers for Medicare and Medicaid Services (CMS)

THERE ARE TIMES when being an interim appointee can be empowering. It may not be particularly dignifying to be considered a "placeholder" while shouldering the extra duties that accompany an interim role, often in addition to your existing job. It can be onerous, to say the least. In that scenario, interim appointees may consider themselves trapped in their circumstances or choose to take a different path. I prefer, as author Ryan Holiday (2014) writes, to let the obstacle become the fuel to create transformation.

Delaware Valley ACO (DVACO) has been around since 2014 and has participated in the Medicare Shared Savings Program (MSSP) for all that time. Over the years, the organization began working more closely with commercial and Medicare Advantage payers in an effort to grow and expand the mission of value-based care. Unfortunately, as the literature suggests, large, hospital-owned MSSPs are less likely to succeed in their efforts to attain shared savings. Despite exceptional leadership and guidance, DVACO was not an outlier in that statistic.

I joined DVACO as the chief medical officer in 2019. Through a unique series of events, including the resignation of our beloved former CEO, by the end of my first year I was asked to become the interim president and CEO of the organization. That request from our board co-chairs felt like an opportunity for personal development as well as a chance to engage our stakeholding health system leaders in a dialogue I knew had to happen. My years of palliative medicine practice had prepared me well to have difficult conversations about the partnership and our overarching goals. Was it time to put the program on life support or hospice?

In summer 2020, amidst the turmoil of the pandemic and civil unrest, I was fortunate enough to engage the leadership at our parent health systems in a dialogue about organizational strategy. What are our true strengths? What are the areas in which we are still developing? What would we need to boost performance in those areas? I am happy to report that the quality performance across the organization has always been excellent. What we needed was a concerted effort by all stakeholders to approach their populations in a more purposeful way. This included managing chronic illness and focusing on a new way of engaging our attributed beneficiaries.

And we needed a partner—one with demonstrated expertise in value-based care. We needed a partner with the financial discipline to evaluate programs with the expert scrutiny that comes from decades of focus in this area. That partner had to be empowered to hold us accountable to our goals and to help us deliver on our mission—to be a part of the solution to serve the community through high-quality, efficient care. That partner would need to be a payer.

CREATING A PATH FOR COLLABORATION

In the fee-for-service ecosystem that persisted for so long, payers and providers were largely siloed from one another. As we know in the healthcare industry, and in most other industries for that matter, silos breed misunderstanding and mistrust. Payers were often made out to be the evil empire by providers, and payers often saw providers as greedily delivering services for personal gain. Neither of those viewpoints is accurate. Providers want to deliver the best possible care driven by the medical literature and yielding the best quality and outcomes for their patients. Payers also want exceptional quality and outcomes and care delivery using solid, evidence-based processes.

There's a nexus there. And an opportunity.

As we know from quality improvement efforts, it is nearly always the systems, rather than the people, that are responsible for less-than-preferable outcomes. Therefore, in this chapter I will look at a change in the system that is becoming more prevalent—the "payvider" ("payer" plus "provider") relationship. In these arrangements, payers and healthcare providers—including medical groups, hospitals, and health systems—collaborate to provide superior care for a population through better outcomes at a lower cost.

In chapter 4, we highlighted accountable care organizations (ACOs). A majority of ACOs operate under some type of payer–provider collaborative arrangement. Because I lead an ACO that is on the higher end of complexity when it comes to these arrangements, I am familiar with the various levels of commitment to these relationships and what they mean. The best way to explain why payvider relationships have grown is to explore why, in value-based care, providers need payers and payers need providers.

WHY DO PROVIDERS NEED PAYERS AND VICE VERSA?

A simplified explanation for why payers and providers need each other is that each group is expert in their own areas and that to thrive we need top performance in multiple areas. Payers know *what* needs to be done to succeed. Providers know *how* to deliver that care.

Additionally, providers bring to the table their relationships with their patients, other network providers, and the community, whereas payers have a well-honed eye for health plan benefit design and an understanding of where inefficiencies, such as wasteful or duplicated spending, may exist.

At DVACO, we have a number of payer programs, and under those payer programs certain elements are easy to accomplish while others are more difficult to achieve. From the provider perspective, collaborating with a payer helps us gain a clearer view of these more challenging elements and gives us a greater understanding of which activities are necessary to accomplish them. Our unique payvider arrangement with Humana also endows the organization with another level of accountability for transforming practice.

Succeeding in value-based care is all about good outcomes. For example, in Medicare Advantage, good performance in the CMS star rating system is foundational. This rating system measures quality performance based on the most current evidence-guided practice. The major domain for Medicare star performance includes quality from the Health Effectiveness Data and Information Set (HEDIS). These ratings account for measures such as cholesterol management in the setting of coronary disease, blood pressure control, and diabetes control.

If an organization receives excellent star ratings, the associated Medicare Advantage program will be well funded by CMS. In contrast, if a star rating drops too low, the program may not be financially viable at all. Star performance is measured on a five-point scale, and a Medicare Advantage program must achieve three and a half stars or better to succeed financially. Under this methodology, payers tend to have the best understanding of the rubric for success while providers are the ones who actually produce outcomes. As a result, when physicians work more closely with payers, we have a better understanding of and focus on the elements of good performance, and this helps us as providers to be better performers.

Similarly, payers need to work with providers because payers don't have the ability to affect certain elements unless they have providers working with them. A prime example is patient experience, which is an important part of good performance. Payers need providers to deliver an exceptional patient experience as part of a total CMS star rating. Suboptimal patient experience not only is bad for patient care; it also reflects poorly on Medicare Advantage programs from the vantage point of both revenue and outcomes.

Finally, payers need providers to drive certain prescribing behaviors. For example, payers will do better in their financial and star-rating performance if their members with diabetes have better outcomes. A payer relies on a provider to perform well in intensive diabetes management and to use drugs (generics whenever possible) that are supported by evidence-based practice to get the most appropriate long-term blood sugar control. This is an example of the provider doing what is best for the patient while at the same time being a good steward of financial resources. (There are several other outcome measurements and standards that are important to both payers and providers in Medicare Advantage and in other programs, and I will cover those in detail in chapter 9 when I present a model for population health.)

THE EVOLUTION OF THE PAYVIDER ARRANGEMENT

Each healthcare market has specific needs. Needs that may emerge include quality performance opportunities, unbridled costs, lagging patient access to care, and more. At times, a provider may see an opportunity to improve care but may not have the capital to move forward. A payer may see an opportunity to grow in a market but may not have the relationships in a given locale to really move the needle. Collaboration affords an opportunity for better outcomes for the community as well as for the providers and the payer.

In many cases the driver of a relationship can be one entity. For example, in an area that is underpenetrated by Medicare Advantage, a Medicare Advantage payer may wish to partner with a provider organization for the opportunity to grow. A provider may wish to partner with a payer when there is an opportunity to better manage a population and to allow the providers an opportunity to achieve a shared-savings arrangement to support their ongoing efforts to transform practice. I recall one particular provider organization coming to me to assist with building its payvider relationship. Its claim was clear: "We are already doing the work and delivering top-notch care. We might as well get paid for it."

Payvider relationships usually evolve over time, rarely jumping into a true payvider ownership arrangement at the start. In our case, DVACO was owned by two provider organizations, Jefferson Health and Main Line Health. In 2022, Humana entered into a joint venture with the organizations as a third equity partner in DVACO and continues as the majority stakeholder as of this writing in 2023.

Indeed, these relationships can assume various configurations to meet the needs of the community. At DVACO, for example, we formed our payvider relationship into a large multipayer, payer-agnostic, risk-bearing entity. That's a mouthful, but basically, as a risk-bearing entity we are an organization that bears risk for providers in order to get rewards that are shared between DVACO and the providers. We incur the bulk of the risk of downside payments and pay a reward to our providers based on a complex algorithm that considers quality, citizenship, and resource stewardship. Although we are majority-owned by Humana, as I noted earlier, we have deep relationships with other national and regional private and governmental payers.

TYPES OF PAYVIDER RELATIONSHIPS

There is some disagreement in the industry about the many types of risk-sharing arrangements in place today among payers and providers. To be clear, not all payvider organizations are universally successful. Considering the possible configurations, I would say there are six distinct collaboration options, which exist on a continuum (see exhibit 5.1). They range from a relatively simple risk-sharing contract to the full joint venture where the payer employs the providers or, as in the case of DVACO, the provider has an ownership stake in the value-based organization.

It is unusual for payer or provider organizations to just dive right into the more intense levels of a payvider arrangement. Typically, the evolution starts near the beginning of this continuum and may take years of learning and problem-solving to advance.

Payer–provider relationships start with fee-for service agreements for services delivered. This arrangement may evolve over time to include fee-for-service reimbursement plus a payment augmentation in which the provider gets extra funding for performing certain quality activities. Eventually, that payment augmentation will begin to move toward actual quality outcomes.

Exhibit 5.1. Risk-Sharing Relationships

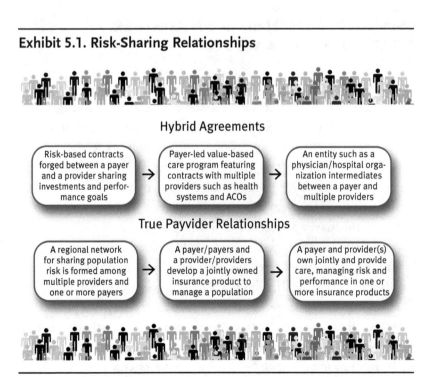

Hybrid Agreements

| Risk-based contracts forged between a payer and a provider sharing investments and performance goals | → | Payer-led value-based care program featuring contracts with multiple providers such as health systems and ACOs | → | An entity such as a physician/hospital organization intermediates between a payer and multiple providers |

True Payvider Relationships

| A regional network for sharing population risk is formed among multiple providers and one or more payers | → | A payer/payers and a provider/providers develop a jointly owned insurance product to manage a population | → | A payer and provider(s) own jointly and provide care, managing risk and performance in one or more insurance products |

Financial performance is also a key part of the value equation in these arrangements. As relationships continue to evolve, the next logical progression includes a shared-savings scenario (which I outlined in chapter 4), in which the total cost of care is managed by both the payer and provider. Remember that in this kind of relationship, if the provider reduces the total cost of care, then the provider gets to participate in a larger percentage of the patient's premium or a larger shared savings.

Moving along the continuum, organizations eventually move into a true payvider relationship. Payvider relationships can take a few different forms. Some payviders will create a collaborative product, which is where the provider organization works directly with the payer to deliver a jointly marketed and administered plan to be offered by employers to their constituents. Joint products can also be a Medicaid or a Medicare Advantage offering.

USING THE DVACO/HUMANA PAYVIDER RELATIONSHIP AS A MODEL

Humana, a well-known and successful Fortune 100 company, is known for its expertise in value-based care for seniors and carries a deep understanding of the complexities and finances of value-based contracting. Provider organizations should not be expected to have that level of expertise at such a granular level. These insights into contracting and payer relations offer opportunities for provider organizations to level up their performance.

As a multipayer organization holding several types of risk contracts, DVACO is among the largest value-based care organizations in the industry. We bring together two key health systems and collaborative partners in the highly competitive greater Philadelphia region into a large, clinically integrated network that provides excellent care with attention to patient experience, access, and outcomes. In partnership with practice leaders in the region, we have demonstrated the ability to make changes in areas that need attention while fostering a learning culture with a focus on resource stewardship.

Like all physicians, participating providers in DVACO want to have adequate time and resources to manage their patients and produce high-quality outcomes. Our physicians and other providers should be paid for the work they are doing and rewarded for quality outcomes. That should be part of their incentive package. Close alignment with a payer allows us to unlock the next level of reward because we bear that higher level of risk. Our experience has been that having strong relationships with multiple regional payers makes us more appealing to other payers, given the knowledge that there is a clear focus on performance.

Across the panoply of payer programs, one theme reigns supreme—payers rely on providers for managing populations with attention to cost while producing the highest-quality outcomes. Much like those mentioned previously, these outcomes within DVACO include appropriate delivery of preventive medicine, such as cancer screenings or vaccinations; chronic disease management; wellness focus; appropriate illness burden documentation; addressing social drivers of health; and patient experience.

Given its unique configuration, DVACO creates safeguards to protect patient information as well as proprietary payer information. It takes a high degree of trust and relationship capital to manage these arrangements well. For this relationship to be successful longitudinally, it is imperative to reach across the aisle, find common ground, and work to achieve it. Silos begone. Our payvider relationship benefits payers, providers, and most importantly, our patients.

PAYVIDER RELATIONSHIPS: HELPING FINANCIAL RISK CONCERNS ON BOTH SIDES

Most providers begin to worry when we talk about two-sided risk. Physicians don't want to deliver care only to be told at some point in the future that the care they delivered costs too much and that they now must pay back a portion of payments received. Provider organizations tend to run narrow margins, so those margins very quickly become negative when it comes to paying back. If that is the case, some believe that it might be better to forgo participating in value-based payments and just collect on traditional fee-for-service terms. And further, a final adjudication on a payer program takes place significantly after actual care has been delivered. I remember doing an end-of-year adjudication for 2019 that was not resolved until mid-2022. Could you imagine if I had to charge back a portion of those fees? That money is already gone. I could think of no faster way to sour a relationship than to request a payback for a service delivered more than three years earlier.

In a payvider arrangement, providers are now an integral part of a payer organization, and payers are typically experts at understanding and managing two-sided risk. In such an arrangement, more often than not, downside payments from individual providers are handled mainly from the parent company. Projections of quality or financial performance are made early to understand any variations in performance. Now the organization has the ability to course-correct in real time to avoid the risk of a downside payment.

Payvider relationships can also help other population health efforts. Often, payers will address what providers may see as burdensome requests for prior authorizations if the payer can officially recognize the provider as a top performer. Payers can also help educate providers in risk coding and reimbursements where needed. This education includes physicians, nurse practitioners, nurses working in practices, and medical assistants. Education programs also need to include clerical staff so that they understand what needs to be done. Do we need prior authorizations for certain studies? Do we need to have some focus on referrals or whatever else may be needed to help the relationship flow properly?

PAYVIDERS AND THE MARCH
TOWARD VALUE-BASED CARE

There is no question that these relationships help providers with risk. When we have a "joint product" between a payer and a provider, we share in the risk, the reward, the outcomes, and the public perception of what happens in our organizations. In managing that joint product, we get to share in all of those things, and that helps providers feel more comfortable with risk. It is easier to move on to two-sided risk arrangements if you're going hand-in-hand with an organization that has been doing downside risk since its inception, because that is the business payers have traditionally engaged in—the risk associated with losses.

The benefit that comes to the patient/member is that now the organization can have a more purely value-based focus, rather than concentrating on collecting fees for additional services delivered to a patient. It's more about keeping a population healthy. The focus is on health equity, high quality, and the patient experience of care. We limit excessive utilization in these kinds of agreements. Things that add no value begin to be erased.

Value-based care is more about keeping the patient well. Wellness becomes the outcome. So how do you keep a population well? Start by addressing acute issues in a timely and responsible manner. For people who have chronic conditions, keep their conditions controlled, prevent them from ending up in the ED, and give people the opportunity to reach out during after-hours if need be. The ultimate benefit is that the focus is on the patient and the population and on keeping the community well.

ARE ALL PAYVIDER RELATIONSHIPS SUCCESSFUL?

As with any business venture, not all payvider collaborations are instantly successful. It should not be considered a magical formula to have a single entity employ the providers and own the insurance carrier. It could be just as easy, maybe easier, for a single owner entity to manage its healthcare delivery network with one set of people and principals, while leaving its insurance product to be managed by a separate team using traditional insurer tactics.

To achieve success, we really need to address the dedication to changing the paradigm of care. A successful collaboration involves breaking down the wall between the payer and the providers and operating as a new company. Many organizations are not ready for that.

George Renaudin, who is president of Medicare and Medicaid for Humana and a board member of DVACO, outlines some of the characteristics that create and sustain successful payvider collaborations. "When they're working well, they're working toward the same aligned goals," he says. "It's easier for that to happen when you're within one organization and you can remove some friction that otherwise would be in place" (Renaudin 2023).

Referring to his experience at Ochsner Health System, Renaudin says,

> In those days, we had the health plan do all the utilization management, with the thought that that is looking at the cost-effectiveness part of the equation. Let the health plan concentrate on that and let us as the healthcare provider concentrate on the quality. Certainly, the two get intermixed, but that was the thinking: Align the organization to provide the best outcome for the patient and for the member at the same time by saying, "We're going to focus on what we do best, and you focus on what you do best."

THE PAYVIDER'S ROLE IN DATA AND ANALYTICS

Our payvider strategy is all about helping us to understand more about our population to better serve our community. Through our payvider partnership, we have come to understand more of the following:

- What are the risks of our population?
- What are the chronic diseases within our population, and how well are they controlled?
- Are our beneficiaries seeing physicians of whom we may be unaware outside our network?

Our patients are often "snowbirds" and travel from the northeastern part of the country down south in the winter. It becomes imperative to know whether an individual had some flare-up of a chronic condition while away that required hospitalization. Claims information supplied through provider relationships offers providers insights into the patient journey and greater opportunities to close the loop on many of those issues.

Renaudin agrees. He states, "I think interoperability can be achieved even without a payvider relationship, but it's much easier when it's in a payvider relationship where everyone is seeing into the same system."

Generally, payers tend to have laser-focused visibility into those intensive analytics and helping to identify patients according to their risk. We can say that these are the patients who are at the highest risk of experiencing a chronic disease exacerbation or requiring hospitalization. So how do we take the clinical resources that we possess as providers and apply them in an intelligent manner to manage that population, keeping them free of exacerbations and out of the hospital?

Payviders and ACOs must use intensive analytics, improved communication channels, and thoughtful patient outreach to help repair the often disjointed and siloed nature of the healthcare system to create a more resilient continuum of care. In the next chapter, we will explore health information technology and concentrated use of analytics that underpin all of the successful population health and community wellness programs presented in this book.

REFERENCES

Holiday, R. 2014. *The Obstacle Is the Way: The Timeless Art of Turning Trials into Triumph.* New York: Penguin.

Renaudin, G. Interview with author. February 21, 2023.

CHAPTER 6

Intensive Analytics

*Hiding within those mounds of data is the knowledge that could
change the life of a patient or change the world.*
Atul Butte, MD, PhD

SEVERAL YEARS AGO, I had a conversation with a group of podiatrists who were interested in collaborating with our organization. I appreciate what podiatrists do for our population and have great respect for their work. Podiatrists manage our diabetic population with meticulous care and maintain our patients' ability to keep all their toes and keep walking on them. In retrospect, it seems that our podiatry consultants didn't fully appreciate the depth of their contribution to the care of accountable care organization (ACO) patients.

I put together a PowerPoint presentation for my conversation with this large podiatry group, and I started off with a demonstration. We explored several of the medications commonly prescribed by podiatrists. These medications ranged from antifungals to anti-inflammatory medications and antibiotics. I showed them the differences in price in some of the formulations of certain drugs and how the costs can vary widely—by many orders of magnitude—for the same drug. Even ibuprofen and famotidine, two older and commonly used drugs for inflammation and stomach protection, respectively, can vary in price by as much as a hundredfold!

I have been a palliative doc for many years now, and I know the coping mechanisms people experience when presented with difficult news: denial, anger, bargaining, depression, and acceptance. It turns out that the same holds true in data presentations.

There was a lot of chatter among the podiatrists in the room as I projected the costs of commonly prescribed drugs on the screen. Some said how incredible the data was. Others frantically looked up drug prices on their phone apps to try to discredit the information. Virtue signaling rang throughout the room, where one of the docs eventually spoke up: "Who would ever write for these expensive formulations which have no benefit to patients?"

"Well, you guys would," I answered. "And this next slide shows your specific prescribing habits over the past six months for our mutual patients." I had redacted the providers' names while listing their prescribing patterns with what we called low-value, high-cost drugs. The top three offending podiatrists on the list each had racked up thousands of dollars in excess drug spending over the six-month period—all without clinical benefit to patients. No one in the room publicly owned up to their part in the costly prescribing debacle, but they knew, and they knew I did as well. This demonstration was a great way to introduce the concept of resource stewardship and analytics to our partners.

INTENSIVE ANALYTICS: THE DRIVER OF THE VALUE STORY

The presentation above demonstrates an effective way to highlight the critical importance of our ultimate driver of action in population health—intensive analytics. The adage "Numbers don't lie" comes alive in the reactions of those podiatrists in that room. Facts are friendly, and data are either pointing in the direction of value for the patient or they are not. In this book so far, I have identified some major roadblocks in providing value-based care to populations and communities. Intensive analytics is one set of tools that rises above all others in creating innovative solutions to all of these challenges.

In many population health organizations, including the one at which I work, we use data-driven tactics to uncover areas of opportunity for improving the health and care of our community. When we address opportunities in a way that brings value to our patients or community, we specifically call these out as our "value stories." We often use this bevy of stories to help focus the team at the beginning of many of our meetings. Over the years we have acquired a trove of stories from our care coordinators, quality assurance team, practice transformation leaders, social workers, and more.

My favorite value stories involve how members of our care team use data to explore areas of redundancy or excess to streamline the patient experience and help navigate the patient through a serious illness. Some of the stories uncover areas of unmet needs for individuals that require connection with community-based organizations. Many of the value stories have demonstrated savings of thousands of dollars to the patient and the system with high-quality and efficient outcomes.

The common thread of intensive analytics runs through many of the value stories of ACOs and the solutions that have been developed in population health. Some of those success stories involve both serving the patients who sit in front of us during their health visits and also finding those who are not present in our clinics but should be.

A great example involves using analytics to address the all-important issue of health inequities. We discussed this topic in depth in chapter 3. To demonstrate the importance of analytics in solving issues related to health equity, it is instructive to look at a list of sample health equity initiatives that the National Association of ACOs (2021) included in a position paper titled "The Role of ACOs in Addressing Health Equity":

- Targeted outreach using information technology and analytics to identify beneficiaries with unmet needs
- Providing interventions to address identified discrepancies or gaps in populations
- Shifting patients with end-stage renal disease or chronic kidney disease (who are disproportionately Black) to more effective and efficient settings that meet their needs and preferences
- Mapping internet access to identify communities with poor access to Wi-Fi or broadband
- Stratifying admission rates and emergency department (ED) visits by race and ethnicity to identify inequities
- Creating care coordination tools for identifying and contacting high-risk patients across a given population to assess their level of food and housing security and their access to medication therapy management

None of these things happen without intensive analytics and the picture it can reveal.

THE STORIES START WITH DATA

The useful and often powerful stories that intensive analytics tells us begin with data—big data. You may have heard that term and waved it off as hyperbole, but it has real meaning. Big data is called that because it is so voluminous and complex that it is nearly impossible to process using traditional databases and methods. When I think about big data, I think about all the data points that accompany a typical clinical encounter. "Big data" is the catch-all term for the barrage of sights, sounds, and other stimuli that continuously come at us and are typically suppressed by the brain to allow us to concentrate.

Your supermarket gathers big data about you. Retail outlets such as Amazon, Target, and Walmart gather data on your access to their venues, your purchase patterns, and your spending. Outlets use that data to suggest additional purchase items for you as well as to drive inventory management. Like it or not, we all are being watched and managed every day by modern analytic methods.

In accountable care, the big data we analyze to add value is gathered from our population. This data is raw and overwhelming—useless in its native form. It includes a variety of information, such as demographics, health conditions, utilization patterns, blood pressure results, prescription fulfillment, and more. Data analytics comes in as the art and science of managing the data so we can use it to tell a story and gain insights about a patient or a population. Revelations from population health analytics can be used to compel or change certain activities or behavior, helping us make the right thing to do the easy thing to do.

So how do we take that large blob of data and mold it into something useful to increase our understanding and drive our decision-making in healthcare?

Data analytics comes in as the art and science of managing the data so we can use it to tell a story and gain insights about a patient or a population.

UNDERSTANDING: A TWO-WAY PROPOSITION

An infrastructure for data and intensive analytics should provide us with a platform that helps us with insights into our patients and populations. In our quest to understand the story of what is happening with our patients, we work to gather information from what I call "the four pillars of population insight": provider-reported data, patient-generated data, health information exchange, and medical claims data (see exhibit 6.1).

Exhibit 6.1. Four Pillars of Population Insight

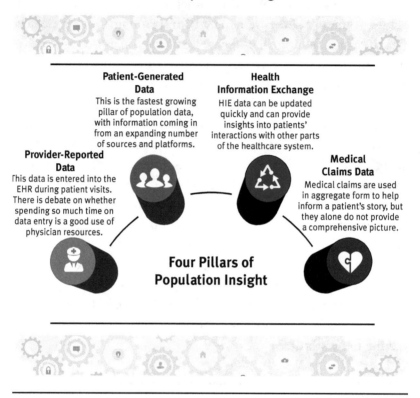

Patient-Generated Data
This is the fastest growing pillar of population data, with information coming in from an expanding number of sources and platforms.

Health Information Exchange
HIE data can be updated quickly and can provide insights into patients' interactions with other parts of the healthcare system.

Provider-Reported Data
This data is entered into the EHR during patient visits. There is debate on whether spending so much time on data entry is a good use of physician resources.

Medical Claims Data
Medical claims are used in aggregate form to help inform a patient's story, but they alone do not provide a comprehensive picture.

Four Pillars of Population Insight

Provider-Reported Data

This is what most individuals would know as the electronic medical record or the more inclusive term, electronic health record (EHR). Providers often ask questions or make observations when a patient is under their care. Those data elements are entered into a provider note for the encounter. Provider notes have been the backbone of fee-for-service billing in the United States for decades now. There is debate over whether it is a good use of physician efforts to spend so much time on data entry during a patient encounter. I think most physicians would argue it is not of benefit.

Patient-Generated Data

Patient-generated data is any information that is provided by the patient. Patient-generated data is the most rapidly growing pillar of population data. Information can come from a variety of sources, from the health history/assessment forms filled out by patients all the way up to in-home remote monitoring technology. Other examples of patient-generated data include the Apple Health app, the Fitbit tracker, continuous blood-glucose monitors, or even more traditional home-based monitoring equipment. Individuals may be tracking their diet or checking their blood pressure, weight, or other measurements at home. In some instances, patients gather this data on their phones and transmit it to their providers. While this data is valuable in helping providers guide care for chronic conditions, it is often voluminous and can require an inordinate amount of provider time to review.

Health Information Exchange

A health information exchange (HIE) is a subscription service that allows me, as a provider, to have access to information about when my patient, for example, goes to the hospital outside my network or to the nursing home across the street. HIE data is quick and can be updated daily. Without HIE data I don't have information about my patient's interactions with other parts of the healthcare system outside of my EHR. HIEs are often geographic in nature.

Medical Claims Data

I admit that I have a love-hate relationship with medical claims.

We can use claims in aggregate form so that they help us inform a patient's story. Consider an example in which I see my patient at my home hospital in Philadelphia. If my patient sees another provider in the same system, I have the data on that visit and can use it to help inform my management of that individual. That is great news. If that same patient, however, has an acute event that requires medical care while traveling with a friend in Chicago, the only way I may be alerted about that event is through a claim. A billing claim will tell me that the patient presented to an ED, was admitted with a specific diagnosis, and had a brief stay. Claims can also provide evidence of a mammogram or other procedure, giving us important information as a fail-safe.

Medical claims are not created to tell a patient's story; they are created for billing purposes. While claims can augment other data, we must use caution because claims are not meant to be a comprehensive picture of the patient's story. Using the traveler example above, if that patient has a CT scan and an MRI while in the hospital, that may be part of the bundled services and not called out in the claims. Results of studies are not typically found in claims either.

Another problem with reliance on claims is that the lag in performance from payers can be massive. Bills can be delayed in any number of areas—at the level of the provider, the billing company, the payer, some rejection process requiring rebilling, and more. In some of our programs we can experience delays of 12 months or more for aggregated claims to find out whether a program is successful in decreasing the cost of care. That makes the learning cycle difficult. As a colleague of mine once said, "Imagine that you are trying to learn to play basketball. You will logically start by shooting some baskets. Now imagine you don't know if those attempts went in the hoop for 12 or more months. It makes for a very slow and inefficient learning cycle."

Yes, it is difficult to learn or do process improvement that way.

GATHERING PATIENT DATA: "WHY DO YOU NEED THIS INFORMATION ABOUT ME?"

Earlier I outlined our four pillars of population insight that help piece together a patient's story. Stories are important, and they help us better understand and manage care of the individual and the population. As it turns out, though, patients are often shielded from the hurdles of data management and may make assumptions about what their providers know. Making such assumptions can lead to poor outcomes.

In population health, we strive to know the patient's journey so that we know where resources are needed and where things are working well. Remember, a large part of population health management is understanding the data about not just the patient in front of me but also the patient who *should be* in front of me. Taking in patients' data and completing their stories using the four pillars helps us to know crucial information about our population in accountable care.

Many beneficiaries participate in a value-based arrangement through their employer relationship with a commercial payer, Medicare, Medicare Advantage, or Medicaid and aren't even aware of what a value-based arrangement is or what that means to them. Beneficiaries may not realize the benefits to them.

We—the individuals running programs of population health and accountable care—have done a poor job of explaining to the consumer the value proposition for their participation in this type of arrangement. Value-based care works best when the patient is engaged. With patient engagement, we have all aspects of care covered.

A large part of population health management is understanding the data about not just the patient in front of me but also the patient who should be in front of me.

Many years ago, a patient asked me to "just tell me when I am due to have my statin prescription refilled." At the time, that seemed like a silly request. I told him that I had a lot of patients and would rely on him to tell me or call his pharmacy when he was running low on pills.

Today, we are aware of critical medication refills, and in the world of value-based care, our quality reimbursements are based on these outcomes. Yes, we now can analyze patients' medication utilization patterns, and they may receive a call or a text to keep them on the right track.

Beneficiaries should understand that the high-tech, high-touch nature of value-based care that they are now receiving exists for reasons other than maximizing trips to the doctor. Through these efforts we are striving for better quality and outcomes, tighter care coordination for complex diseases, fewer repetitive and unnecessary tests, a focus on evidence-based protocols in medicine, exploration and adherence to patient goals, and care delivery that meets their specific needs in the community where they live and work. Now this is why I went into medicine!

THE ROLE OF ANALYTICS IN POPULATION HEALTH AND VALUE-BASED CARE

In writing this book I interviewed Aneesh Chopra, CEO of Care-Journey, a large data aggregator and analytics warehouse. He was appointed by President Barack Obama as the first Chief Technology Officer of the United States (2009 to 2012). Prior to that, Chopra served as Virginia's secretary of technology under Governor Tim Kaine. He illustrated the contrast of how we in healthcare use health information technology in a fee-for-service environment compared to value-based care:

In the fee-for-service world, the job we give software is to improve scheduling optimization to ensure there are no empty slots, to accurately document the severity of a visit to improve revenue capture, to execute payment transactions and follow-up so you get paid your fair share in a timely manner, and to minimize administrative burden in executing on all three of those things. The productivity function is very clear in fee-for-service, and frankly, a lot of money has been spent on improving those three things.

In value-based care, it is much more about forecasting and analytics to determine which individuals you should engage on the assumption that they may need help. Avoidable, unplanned admissions and ED visits remain the "never-events" objective for reduction. So having much more up-front investment on care plans, understanding the patient conditions and needs, monitoring their medications, staying active—all of those steps require technology to ingest more information about the patient, to analyze it, to rejigger the sorting list for where to prioritize the outreach. (Chopra 2022)

TURNING THE DATA FROM RAW TO COOKED

Healthcare data can point to important usage patterns when analyzed properly. For instance, we have found that about 45 percent of ED usage happens during typical business hours (Monday through Friday, 8 a.m. to 5 p.m.) and that another 25 percent happens on the weekends. Why is it important to explore usage patterns? Well, perhaps that means that primary doctors in the area don't have adequate access on weekends. Or it may be that the patients are coming in from nursing homes on days when the facilities are typically understaffed. Data analysis helps us make evidence-guided decisions to address the care of the population in ways that are most meaningful.

After a recent board presentation our team made showing opportunities in the region, I received a call from the CEO of one of the local health systems. He said, "I love the way this data is presented. I want to take a deeper dive into the data specific to my health system. We have experienced a significant uptick in ED utilization, and the system is struggling to handle the higher volume of patients. How can we explore the root of the changes to improve capacity for those who truly need the services?" I brought this inquiry to our analytics team to explore. How do we understand the patients presenting to the ED while exploring what fraction of them are better suited to be managed in the outpatient offices? And if we can manage them in the primary care setting, what are the workloads we would need to address in this series of what are called "ambulatory-sensitive conditions"? This is all in a day's work in value-based care.

Another problem we frequently encounter is the administration of certain high-cost drugs in the ambulatory setting. To be clear, when a high-cost drug is the right (or only) option, we support its use to improve the lives of our beneficiaries. In a setting where a lower-cost alternative may offer a similar or even better therapeutic option, we work with our providers to understand their drug choice. These conversations tend to be highly sensitive. Keeping in mind that facts are friendly, comparative data help facilitate a discussion.

Often, we will collect data for a given specialty using multiple practices in the area as comparators. We will then be able to make comparisons regarding cost or outcomes. Exhibit 6.2 shows how we use visual analytics to tell the story of how various practices perform on cost. Each circle represents a practice, and the size of the circle represents the size of the practice. In this example, we find that Practice C is a negative outlier when it comes to cost of care. And no one wants to be the outlier.

Physicians and other types of providers in value-based care are often the stewards of resources. Unfortunately, providers are often blind to the costs of their tests and treatments. The American health system is incredibly strange in that regard. Providers do not know the cost of what they prescribe, and patients—when insured—are often shielded from cost as well. That leaves us with a system where

Exhibit 6.2. Cost of Care by Provider

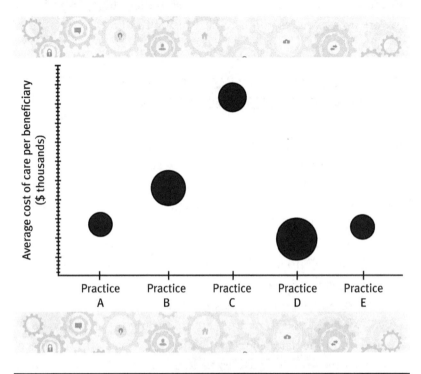

only the payer is actually informed about what healthcare costs. I can think of no other industry where such a dynamic exists.

Here is a thought experiment. Imagine you are going to purchase a new car. You probably want the best car to meet your needs. It should be safe, efficient, reliable, and stylish. What if someone else picked the car for you based on your needs? Now imagine that neither of you know anything about what the vehicle costs, and neither of you have to bear the brunt of the cost. I don't see a ton of incentive to be cost-conscious in that scenario.

My pharmacology instructor in medical school once said, "Your pen is the most dangerous and costly instrument you will use in medicine." Nearly 30 years later, the pen has been replaced by the keyboard in that conversation, but the statement still rings true. Providers must be made aware of the cost of their therapies and tests if we are ever to create good stewardship of resources.

USING ALTERNATIVE PAYMENT MODELS FOR ORGANIZATIONAL INCENTIVES

Another example of using intensive analytics to influence behavior is with organizational behavior. Some newer value-based programs, such as ACO REACH (Realizing Equity, Access, and Community Health), have structures that provide opportunities for influencing behavior. The ACO REACH model will allow ACOs to directly contract with a specific acute-care hospital or perhaps even a skilled nursing facility (SNF) to deliver high-quality and cost-conscious care.

This means that if I am working in an ACO, I can use intensive analytics to see where my costs are. Then I can approach an SNF to say, "We need you to deliver care that is high-quality and cost-conscious, and the data tell us that we are more cost-effective when we keep people for *as long as they need*, not *as long as their insurance will pay*."

With that, ACOs and other organizations can enter into an agreement together, and everyone shares the risk. The SNF now has the opportunity to say, "We're not going to keep this patient for 21 days just because their insurance will pay for it. Wouldn't it be great if we delivered care in only seven days and then spent three more days developing an appropriate transition-to-home plan? We could focus on helping the patient get in and out of the car, up their steps, and back into their home." That's probably the better way to do it rather than having the patient stay at the SNF for the maximum allowable days.

USING INTENSIVE ANALYTICS TO
IMPROVE THE PATIENT EXPERIENCE

In value-based organizations, we analyze payer data on many different levels. For example, we use data from payers to help us understand things like care gaps. A care gap can be defined as any lapse in adherence to evidence-based practice, such as mammograms, colonoscopies, or blood sugar control in the setting of diabetes. All that information comes together to make up our Medicare Advantage star rating as explained in chapter 5. The higher the star rating on the five-point scale, the better the quality of an organization. And as we have already discussed in this book, in the world of value-based care, strong performance on quality equals better outcomes. These outcomes are better for patients and better for finances.

In writing this book, I interviewed Cori McMahon, PsyD, chief clinical officer at ERP Health and former vice president of clinical services for Tridiuum, now known as Lucet. A psychologist and leader in the field of behavioral health, she is also an associate professor of clinical medicine at Cooper Medical School at Rowan University in Camden, New Jersey. She related to me the following example of a common situation that can be remedied by intensive analytics:

> A good tech platform can improve the patient and provider experience from the patient's first connection with healthcare. Think about the very common scenario in which a patient is seeking behavioral healthcare and makes a phone call to the number on their insurance card. They get a person on the line who asks them a few questions to understand what their geographic region is and what their issue might be. What they will usually get next is either an e-mail or a hard copy in the mail with a list of 20 or so providers. (McMahon 2022)

Dr. McMahon pointed out that the problem is that these lists often have not been vetted for being current or accurate. "We don't know if the providers are the right fit, or have the necessary expertise, or are even taking new patients," she said. "In a large amount of the cases, the patient never gets connected with a provider. They also have to go through the disappointing and sometimes grueling experience of making phone call after phone call that goes nowhere."

Additionally, Dr. McMahon noted that mental health providers are often heavily booked or are lacking in administrative support, so they are not able to follow up on phone calls. She said that because of her other academic and corporate commitments at one point, she was only doing mental health clinical work part-time in an HIV clinic. However, she still received weekly phone calls from patients referred by their insurance carrier who, for example, were looking for care for their child who is on the autism spectrum or for other conditions that were completely outside of her current area of focus. She was on the call list because she was a behavioral health clinician and she was geographically close to the person for whom the list was generated.

"I would still try to help the patient find an appropriate provider, but that is not usually the case for most people seeking care," McMahon said. She then provided an example of what happens when intensive analytics are being used in a call center:

> It can do a couple of things. It can aggregate and surface all of the availability in real time for providers who are participating and willing to put their schedules in, and it can also do a better job of matching a patient with a best-fit provider. So if you have done a quick assessment with a patient on the phone, or better yet, you have used technology to do that, you can get a sense of the main presenting problem—maybe it's depression or post-traumatic stress or substance abuse—and then the technology can filter in the right providers and surface them. Then you can make that connection on that same phone call

and actually get that patient scheduled. So this is a completely different patient experience.

MOVING FORWARD WITH INTENSIVE ANALYTICS

One thing that is immediately apparent is that none of the programs we have highlighted in this chapter would ever get off the ground without a deeper level of understanding about the population. For success in value-based care, you need information from patients, EHRs, claims data, and health system information technology infrastructure. This requires commitment and resources from the organizations involved, but the outcome is worthwhile. If we plan to manage the health of our communities, we cannot do it without such commitment.

A joint study from Humana and the Medical Group Management Association (MGMA), released in fall 2022, addressed the importance of value-based care in the momentum toward intensive analytics:

> The healthcare industry has spent years talking about moving toward interoperability and improved data sharing among practices, patients, and payers. While there remains a long way to go to achieve true interoperability, the adoption of value-based care arrangements is bringing more medical groups up to speed with the types of IT tools needed to collect, measure and report quality metrics. (MGMA and Humana 2022, 9)

The Humana/MGMA study found that the top technological additions to those provider organizations that were related to improving their value-based care arrangement participation were data analytics and reporting platforms, population health management tools, and EHRs. The top three paid resources committed by the organizations to help with the move toward value-based care were staff, technology, and patient engagement. The primary types of staff added were in care coordination, care management, and data analytics.

Much of this chapter highlights the value of and need for cooperation between payers and provider organizations in sharing information. Humana and MGMA teaming up for the aforementioned study is an example of such cooperation. Humana has entered into value-based partnerships with multiple organizations across the country, including the one in which I serve. In that collaborative approach we share not only information among providers and payers but also the financial risk of serving a population's health needs while improving both financial and health outcomes. That is the payvider arrangement we presented in chapter 5.

In the next chapter we will continue to explore analytics, and how they combine with audacious initiatives to address closing gaps in our population health and community wellness efforts—particularly in behavioral health and palliative care.

REFERENCES

Chopra, A. Interview with author. November 23, 2022.

McMahon, C. Interview with author. November 10, 2022.

Medical Group Management Association (MGMA) and Humana. 2022. *Shifting to Value amid Pandemic and Staffing Challenges: MGMA and Humana Joint Research Study Report.* Published September 22. http://mgma.com/practice-resources/revenue-cycle/shifting-to-value-amid-pandemic-and-staffing-chall.

National Association of ACOs. 2021. "The Role of ACOs in Addressing Health Equity." Published September 21. http://naacos.com/assets/docs/pdf/2021/ACOsandHealthEquity-PositionPaper092121.pdf.

CHAPTER 7

Behavioral Health and Palliative Care: Uncovering Unmet Needs

What mental health needs is more sunlight, more candor, and more unashamed conversation.
Glenn Close

FLOYD WAS A 69-year-old man with poorly controlled diabetes who lived alone. His journey with serious illness started when he first noticed his eyes turning yellow along with feelings of lethargy and abdominal discomfort. Upon presentation to the emergency department, he was noted to have gallstones. An adept resident physician found that his degree of liver failure went beyond an impacted stone; upon further examination, she uncovered his ongoing alcohol consumption. Floyd then experienced a prolonged hospital stay where he received supportive care while waiting for his liver function to return on its own. Eventually, he was able to undergo an endoscopic procedure to remove the stone, and with instructions to avoid alcohol, he was sent to a short-term rehab facility.

Floyd's course in rehab was particularly tumultuous and culminated in a reprimand for drinking alcohol, which his friend snuck in for him. The facility agreed to allow him to finish his stay with the caveat that he would not drink while he was recuperating. Floyd completed the last five days of his stay while secretly continuing his surreptitious alcohol consumption.

Upon discharge, Floyd quickly resumed even heavier alcohol consumption. By his 11th day home, he was again jaundiced, and his legs and abdomen were filling up with fluid. He decided to go to a different hospital this time because of "disagreements" with the nursing staff during his original stay. His second hospitalization was more than three weeks long and filled with a repeat of much of the same workup that was done at the original facility.

When physicians determined he was "about as good as he will get," a discharge planner suggested rehab—a suggestion he violently refused. He wanted to go home. He was given a prescription for his worsening liver failure, which he never filled upon discharge. At this point Floyd became what we call *lost to follow-up.*

His story came to an unfortunate ending when he was helicoptered to an area tertiary care center (now his third hospital) with fulminant liver failure. He was placed in the intensive care unit, where he required mechanical ventilation and high-dose intravenous medications to elevate his dropping blood pressure. Family members were unable to be reached to help with his medical decision-making. Typically, when no decision-maker is available, the default decision is for full aggressive measures. When his heart finally gave out, he died a somewhat brutal death as he received three rounds of CPR late one evening with chest compressions and multiple unsuccessful attempts to revive him.

His was a very difficult ending I will not forget.

A SORRY STATE OF AFFAIRS

Floyd is not alone.

Among the 138.5 million people in the United States who were alcohol users in 2020, 61.6 million of them (or 44.4 percent) were binge drinkers over the previous month (defined as "current use"). Among those current alcohol users, 17.7 million were current heavy drinkers. And those are just the numbers regarding alcohol, according to the US Substance Abuse and Mental Health Services

Administration (SAMHSA) 2021 annual report. That report also notes that in 2020, 58.7 percent of the population—162.5 million people—were current users of tobacco, alcohol, or illicit drugs. And as in Floyd's case, substance use disorder represents just a fraction of maladaptive mental health conditions.

In the same report, SAMHSA noted that in 2020 more than one in five adults—52.9 million people—in the United States lived with some form of mental illness, and 5.6 percent—over 14 million people—had serious mental illness.

These statistics highlight a considerable segment of our population who, to improve or even immediately save their lives, need care along a continuum from minor lifestyle modification to aggressive behavioral health interventions. The bad news is that the healthcare system generally does not do a good job of identifying these people in the community and getting them the help they need.

SICK AND TIRED OF BEING SICK AND TIRED

In the United States, so many aspects of behavioral and emotional health are simply not addressed as doctors steer focus toward the pathophysiology of disease. It certainly is a lot cleaner to focus our efforts on the mechanical aspects of the body than to dive into emotional aspects such as depression, anxiety, loneliness, or isolation. In reality, physical and emotional conditions coexist the vast majority of the time. Not only does chronic illness often precipitate depression, anxiety, and other forms of emotional instability, but the converse is also true.

Let's look at how this might happen. For example, someone is diagnosed with a chronic illness such as heart failure. That patient will be affected by the fear of knowing that this diagnosis will affect their ability to function independently in life. A diagnosis of heart disease can create anxiety over taking a walk, a swim, or even a trip to the supermarket. Fears will logically arise about the likelihood of ongoing symptoms, heavy medication burden, the cost of care, and even the possibility of shortened life expectancy. "How is heart failure going to impact me financially? How is this going to affect my significant other and my children? Who will care for me if I cannot care for my own basic needs?"

According to the National Institute of Mental Health (NIMH), having a chronic illness increases the likelihood of developing a mental health condition. One mental health condition in particular—depression—is particularly common among people who have chronic illnesses, including

- Alzheimer's disease;
- autoimmune diseases such as systemic lupus erythematosus, rheumatoid arthritis, and psoriasis;
- cancer;
- heart disease;
- diabetes;
- epilepsy;
- HIV/AIDS;
- hypothyroidism;
- multiple sclerosis;
- Parkinson's disease; and
- stroke and stroke-related conditions (NIMH 2021a).

As in the example above, if someone has been diagnosed with heart disease and they suddenly find themselves limited in doing activities that used to bring them joy, symptoms of depression may begin to emerge.

This cause-and-effect association between chronic conditions and depression and anxiety can also go the other way. In one study of more than 40,000 people in three age groups, women with depression and comorbid depression/anxiety across all age groups had an increased risk of accumulating chronic medical conditions compared to people without depression and anxiety. This was also true of the younger men in the study (Bobo et al. 2022).

SEEING THE GAPS IS VITAL TO BRIDGING THEM

The effects of chronic illness are as deep as they are broad. As we manage the members within our populations, we must be mindful that mental health disorders are likely present along with chronic physical health conditions as either effects or contributory causes. Given the constraints of the system in American medicine, we often fail to focus on the behavioral aspects of care in chronic illness management. A clear-cut connection exists between people's chronic illnesses and their mental health, and we don't do an especially good job of identifying this and then helping patients through it.

Given the constraints of the system in American medicine, we often fail to focus on the behavioral aspects of care in chronic illness management.

The numbers bear that out. Among 11 high-income countries across the globe, the United States has the highest rate of adults (23 percent) who report having a mental health diagnosis. At the same time, the United States also reports some of the worst outcomes related to mental health among those countries, including the second-highest rate of death due to drugs and the highest rate of suicide (Tikkanen et al. 2020).

While mental health issues were prevalent before the COVID-19 pandemic, alarmingly, the pandemic made matters even worse. The pandemic demonstrated how the need for behavioral health services is affected by social and environmental factors. Pandemic living brought about a massive outbreak of psychological illness due to factors such as social isolation, limits on businesses, stay-at-home orders, financial pressures, grief, fear of illness and death, unemployment, and food and housing insecurity. A Centers for Disease Control and Prevention study reported that from August 2020 through February 2021, the percentage of adults reporting symptoms of anxiety or depressive disorder increased from 36.4 percent to 41.5 percent—a significant jump during a relatively short period during the height of the pandemic. Those reporting that they needed but did not receive mental health counseling or therapy during the preceding four weeks also increased significantly to 11.7 percent (Vahratian et al. 2021).

As it did with all morbidity and mortality, the pandemic highlighted inequities related to mental health in the population along racial lines as well. When adjusted for age, Black, Hispanic, and American Indian or Alaska Native people experienced higher rates of COVID-19 infection and death than White Americans. The higher infection rates are attributed in part to several social drivers of health, including transportation issues, living in larger households, and working in jobs that could not be performed remotely (Ndugga, Hill, and Artiga 2022).

According to a Kaiser Family Foundation study (Hamel et al. 2020), more than half of adults of all racial and ethnic groups said the pandemic had a negative impact on their emotional health, but Black and Hispanic people were nearly twice as likely as White adults to agree that the pandemic had a "major negative impact."

WHAT DOES BEHAVIORAL HEALTH ENCOMPASS?

In my interview with Dr. Cori McMahon (see chapter 6), she noted that the definition of behavioral healthcare varies, even among people who are engaged in managing and delivering it.

> **Dr. Angelo:** How would you explain the difference between behavioral healthcare and mental healthcare?
> **Dr. McMahon:** I would say behavioral health is a more all-encompassing term as opposed to mental health being more specifically focused on mood functioning or psychological dysfunction in particular.

Behavioral health encompasses psychiatry, psychology, and all of the other specific work that a therapist, social worker, addiction counselor, or other professional would perform.

Dr. Angelo: Even my own understanding of behavioral health has grown over the years. Now I see behavioral health as more of an umbrella term, while mental health involves more specifically addressing mental disorders. I see behavioral health as larger.

Dr. McMahon: Yes, absolutely. In my clinical practice, I would note that behavioral health encompasses the behavioral medicine team, the psychiatry folks, the social workers, and the addictions med team. Behavioral health seems to be described—and I agree—as the larger umbrella term that encompasses something beyond our mood functioning, so behavioral health includes the rest of the gamut, such as substance use, smoking, eating, preventive care, diet and exercise, and the interplay between behavior and health.

BARRIERS TO BEHAVIORAL HEALTH IN POPULATION HEALTH MANAGEMENT

Social stigma around seeking professional mental health services has always been a major barrier to care. One of the areas with the greatest social stigma in behavioral health is suicidal ideation. In a widely cited survey of 2,200 US adults conducted by three national organizations dedicated to suicide prevention, respondents were asked, "What do you think are some of the barriers that prevent people who are thinking about suicide from seeking help?" The top three responses, in order, were *feeling like nothing will help, embarrassment,* and *not knowing how to get help* (Anxiety and Depression Association of America, American Foundation for Suicide Prevention, and Action Alliance for Suicide Prevention 2016).

The differences between college-aged adults (ages 18 to 25) and older adults in this survey are striking. While a greater percentage of college-aged adults said that behavioral health issues were among the top three barriers for them, they were also much more likely to consider seeing a mental health professional "as a sign of strength" compared to the older adults in the survey (60 percent versus 35 percent). Younger people were also more likely to have visited a mental health professional within the past 12 months compared to older adults (18 percent versus 11 percent), even though they were significantly less likely to have seen a primary care physician during the past year.

In addition to social stigma, a significant percentage of respondents cited barriers to seeking behavioral healthcare, including inability to afford treatment, lack of access to treatment, lack of social support, fear of disappointing others, and fear of losing a job. These perceived barriers are common throughout the spectrum of behavioral health management. In case you are not so sure about the lack of access, I encourage you to do your own experiment and try to get a non-emergent behavioral health appointment that is in your community and covered by your insurance. Chances are remarkably high that you will wait months if you are able to get an appointment at all.

BREAKING DOWN THE BARRIERS

Many of these barriers are more than just perception—they are realities. In the United States we suffer a lack of capacity to manage behavioral health, and that perception is amplified by the lack of access to care and inability of so many to afford it. If providers are interested in advancing population health and community wellness, we must increase our involvement in the behavioral aspects of dealing with chronic illness and disability.

One encouraging step in this direction was made in early 2022, when the American Psychological Association (APA), which has more than 121,000 members, developed a policy titled "Psychology's Role in Advancing Population Health." A release announcing the newly adopted policy stated that "psychologists should adopt a population health approach to their work, focusing on the health of entire communities." It continued, "For population health models to be most effective, researchers, practitioners, educators and students of the science of psychology should be actively engaged in the research/development, design, implementation, operation and evaluation of these systems and initiatives" (APA 2022).

"Psychologists should adopt a population health approach to their work, focusing on the health of entire communities."

In its policy the APA laid out four guiding principles for the use of members, committees, divisions, and boards in their population health endeavors:

1. **Work within and across diverse systems to advance population health.** This includes partnering with community leaders, local institutions, faith-based organizations, schools, employers, and others to develop solutions that address the unique challenges of their communities, including available resources and social drivers of health.

2. **Work "upstream" by promoting prevention and early intervention strategies.** Psychologists contribute to developing, disseminating, and implementing evidence-based models for prevention and early intervention and would create tools to screen and monitor for unmet needs.

3. **Educate psychologists and community partners on population health.** This involves educating psychologists and others in the behavioral health workforce in concepts of population health and community wellness, using an equity, diversity, and inclusion approach and focusing on research.

4. **Enlist a diverse array of community partners.** This includes the involvement of a broad range of national, state, and local stakeholders within and outside of health care. (APA 2022)

This sounds like a solid framework for a population health blueprint. Even before this policy was adopted, some ACOs were using all these evidence-based principles to meet behavioral population health objectives. A good example is the following case study presented by the Centers for Medicare & Medicaid Services (CMS) on its Innovation Models website (CMS 2016).

Atrius Health, based in eastern Massachusetts, has been developing and refining its behavioral health program since 2015. This ACO remains a leader in population behavioral health and offers its Behavioral Health Fellowship, which is a one-year, full-time, interdisciplinary program open to postdoctoral psychologists and postgraduate social workers.

A substantial problem before the start of the program was that full-time therapists had average caseloads of more than 100 active patients, which meant they could not see patients more than once per month: well below the once-a-week recommendation in the literature for effective treatment. In addition, new patients had average wait times of 60 days for an initial therapy session and 45 days for follow-up appointments.

The solution had two major elements:

1. A triage and referral process was designed so that behavioral health clinicians saw the most clinically complex patients while high-functioning patients were referred to an external network of community health providers.

2. Evidence-based guidelines were developed, implemented, and trained so that patients in the program received consistent, measurable treatment focused on solutions.

This program has resulted in reduced caseloads for clinicians and significantly decreased wait times for new patients who need services the most. It has also helped ensure that patients are quickly routed to the lowest-cost setting appropriate to their care needs. However, I should point out that while triaging new referrals is an appropriate and timely way to serve patients with the highest needs early, suspending care for patients of any level of need is still unfavorable, especially if you or your loved one is the one in need.

TELEHEALTH AS PART OF THE SOLUTION

The NIMH cites several potential benefits of virtual visits—known as telemental or telebehavioral health in this context—that relate to population health and community wellness considerations presented earlier in this book. Exhibit 7.1 shows some of the major potential benefits.

Of course, as with all types of virtual health services, taking advantage of the opportunities of telebehavioral health in the future depends on continued reimbursement of a wide range of virtual behavioral health services. Realizing the full benefit of telebehavioral health in the future will also require population health efforts to ensure that people disadvantaged by lack of access to devices for virtual visits or to high-speed internet are not falling through the cracks and are able to take advantage of this care modality.

People enter the behavioral health management system generally in one of two ways—either through self-referral or referral by a primary care (or other) provider. The success of the APA policy, the Atrius Health program, and the telebehavioral health solutions described earlier all rely on the referral process. As with other chronic disease management, poor access is the weak link in the chain of managing behavioral health at a population level.

This means that providers of population health must strive to support the primary care relationship while identifying the right

Exhibit 7.1. Potential Benefits of Telebehavioral Health

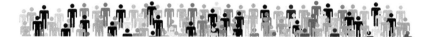

Reaching more people by removing barriers. Virtual health visits make mental health services available to some people who have not previously had access to them, including in emergency situations and in remote locations. Also, the privacy that telebehavioral health affords may be seen as a good option for people who have been reluctant to engage in traditional mental health services.

Addressing social drivers of health with convenience. Issues of lack of transportation, availability of childcare, and limited opportunities to take time off from work may be overcome by using telehealth. Also, people can schedule appointments at more flexible hours and with less notice.

Increasing availability of telebehavioral health. Since the beginning of the pandemic, telebehavioral health services became more widely available as more providers embraced the technology and migrated a greater percentage of their practices permanently to the virtual space.

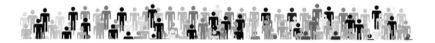

Source: Data from NIMH (2021b).

individuals for referral to behavioral health professionals. We are challenged to do a better job in the community behavioral health arena.

UNDERSTANDING PATIENT NEEDS THROUGH SHARED DECISION-MAKING

Another important aspect of population health and value-based care involves understanding the needs and wishes of the members of a given community. Medicine has historically had a very paternalistic approach to care delivery. The imperatives have been to follow doctors' orders because, of course, "doctor knows best." Consequently, if you failed to follow your doctor's orders, you were labeled "noncompliant," and you were on your own.

I am happy to report that much has changed in recent years, and doctors and other providers have taken a wider view using communication about patient-centered goals. Often, if a patient is found to have a serious illness, the first inclination is to work toward a cure. If a cure cannot be achieved, then the typical desires of the patient and family are to minimize the burden of illness and allow the person to lead their life as they see fit.

It is important not to assume we know the goals of our population. As a rule, when providers ask patients about their goals of care, they can fit into the categories of curative, restorative, or palliative care. And these goals do not exist in a vacuum. Patients may want palliation (meaning relief from suffering) as well as an opportunity to achieve some level of cure. Similarly, individuals who are debilitated from some underlying illness may want to have function restored, as well as comfort.

Shared decision-making requires us not to make assumptions about what an individual wants. Sometimes getting to the bottom of a goals conversation requires us to simply ask, "What are you hoping for from this situation?"

While not all goals may be feasible, it is important to explore and understand the underlying drivers. In some situations, I will ask patients, "What is it that you are most worried about?" The replies are quite often concerns about pain, suffering, losing independence, and being a burden on others.

THE INTERSECTION OF PALLIATIVE CARE AND POPULATION HEALTH

I have had the opportunity to be a palliative physician for many years now, and it has truly been an honor to serve my patients. Palliative care is one of those fields where many people don't really know what

I do. When I am asked at a party what a palliative care doctor is, I tell folks that I take care of seriously ill people and help with pain and symptom management as well as complex decision-making and goals of care. Once I tell people about this type of work, I have learned to anticipate their response: "How could you do that kind of work? Isn't that depressing?"

Yes, my work can be intense, but I have the best job in the whole hospital. I get to meet people when they most need a hand and learn about their lives, their wishes. I get to hear so many amazing stories—stories of hope, stories of love, stories of life in general. So many patients and their families let me into their inner circle for these in-depth, privileged conversations. I witness immense hope and help people confront fears with strength they never knew they had. I prescribe medication and other therapies to alleviate pain and suffering. I help patients and families understand their illness on a deeper level and bring their wishes to fruition. Whose job could be better than that?

There is overlap between the work we do in palliative care and the work of population health. For both areas, we focus on the wishes of the patient, and we strive to deliver patient-centric care. Both palliative care and population health use a team-based approach to deliver services such as therapy, medical equipment, home-based care, and medication reconciliation in a comprehensive manner with an eye on resource stewardship. Neither palliative care nor population health is transactional in nature—we are in it for the long game.

Accordingly, palliative services are an excellent tool for an ACO as well. For instance, home-based palliative care services help patients in their times of need while directing resources where care is most appropriate. In fact, researchers demonstrated that when patients in an ACO receive home-based palliative care, their total cost of care is approximately $12,000 lower than the cost for those who went without the service. The home care group was able to stay in their preferred setting and had about one-third fewer trips to the hospital (Lustbader et al. 2017). When DVACO deployed a similar program for home-based management, we found similar outcomes. This is truly a win from multiple perspectives.

PALLIATIVE CARE IS DELIVERED ALONGSIDE DISEASE-MODIFYING CARE

Palliative care is considered a part of the management of chronic disease. Some patients may need more of a palliative intervention, while others have little need based on symptoms and functionality. Older models of palliative care focused on disease-modifying care until that was no longer feasible, and then a patient would begin to use palliative services. A great deal has changed since then. Exhibit 7.2 shows how we currently view palliative alongside curative services. While the authors initially published this reference in 2015, through iteration it remains as the mainstay of how providers deliver palliative and disease-directed care in concert.

Exhibit 7.2. Palliative Care in Disease Management

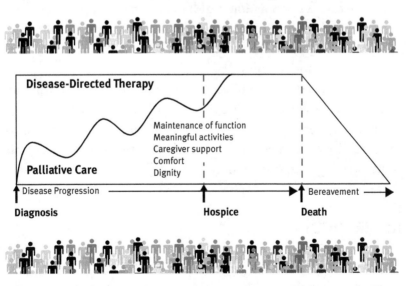

Source: Adapted from Lee et al. (2018).

Palliative care exists on a continuum. It begins with a diagnosis of any serious illness and continues along the entire course of the patient's illness. Sometimes palliative care services culminate in the utilization of hospice care, while at other times patients graduate from a palliative clinic if their underlying illness is controlled and their needs are few.

It was initially thought that although hospice and palliative care improved quality of life, these services would hasten the end of someone's life. To the contrary, studies have shown that patients actually live *longer* when they receive palliative care (Temel et al. 2010; Hoerger et al. 2019). It is believed that this type of care alleviates suffering and allows patients to receive treatments that they and their providers deem appropriate.

EXPANDING CARE BEYOND BEHAVIORAL AND PALLIATIVE CARE

Now that we have explored the benefits of behavioral health and palliative care for population health management, it is evident that the drivers of this type of care should not favor transactional or episodic services. We are in this for the infinite game and must focus on outcomes, not episodes.

This is the perfect time to begin our discussion of the continuum of care and how we deliver comprehensive, team-based, "wraparound" services to manage those with chronic illness and to maximize quality outcomes. In the next chapter we will dive into this topic, starting with care management.

REFERENCES

American Psychological Association (APA). 2022. "APA Calls for Population Health Approach to Solve Critical Issues in

Society." Published March 10. https://www.apa.org/news/press/releases/2022/03/population-health-critical-issues.

Anxiety and Depression Association of America, American Foundation for Suicide Prevention, and Action Alliance for Suicide Prevention. 2016. "A Survey About Mental Health and Suicide in the United States." Published January 14. http://adaa.org/sites/default/files/College-Aged_Adults_Survey_Summary-1.14.16.pdf.

Bobo, W. V., B. R. Grossardt, S. Virani, J. L. St. Sauver, C. M. Boyd, and W. A. Rocca. 2022. "Association of Depression and Anxiety with the Accumulation of Chronic Conditions." *Journal of the American Medical Association Network Open* 5 (5): e229817. http://doi.org/10.1001/jamanetworkopen.2022.9817.

Centers for Medicare and Medicaid Services (CMS). 2016. "Improving Behavioral Health Care for Medicare Beneficiaries: Atrius Health." Published September. http://innovation.cms.gov/files/x/aco-casestudy-atrius.pdf.

Hamel, L., L. Lopes, C. Munana, S. Artiga, and M. Brodie. 2020. *Race, Health, and COVID-19: The Views and Experiences of Black Americans.* Kaiser Family Foundation. Published October 14. http://files.kff.org/attachment/Report-Race-Health-and-COVID-19-The-Views-and-Experiences-of-Black-Americans.pdf.

Hoerger, M., G. R. Wayser, G. Schwing, A. Suzuki, and L. M. Perry. 2019. "Impact of Interdisciplinary Outpatient Specialty Palliative Care on Survival and Quality of Life in Adults with Advanced Cancer: A Meta-Analysis of Randomized Controlled Trials." *Annals of Behavioral Medicine* 53 (7), 674–85.

Lee, E. E., B. Chang, S. Huege, and J. Hirst. 2018. "Complex Clinical Intersection: Palliative Care in Patients with Dementia." *American Journal of Geriatric Psychiatry* 26 (2): 224–34.

Lustbader, D., M. Mudra, C. Romano, E. Lukoski, A. Chang, J. Mittelberger, T. Scherr, and D. Cooper. 2017. "The Impact of a Home-Based Palliative Care Program in an Accountable Care Organization." *Journal of Palliative Medicine* 20(1): 23–28.

National Institute of Mental Health (NIMH). 2021a. "Chronic Illness and Mental Health: Recognizing and Treating Depression." Accessed June 7, 2023. http://nimh.nih.gov/health/publications/chronic-illness-mental-health.

——————.2021b. "What Is Telemental Health?" Washington, DC: National Institutes of Health, Publication No. 21-MH-8155. https://www.nimh.nih.gov/sites/default/files/health/publications/what-is-telemental-health/what-is-telemental-health.pdf.

Ndugga, N., L. Hill, and S. Artiga. 2022. "COVID-19 Cases and Deaths by Race/Ethnicity as of Fall 2022." Kaiser Family Foundation. Published November 17. http://kff.org/coronavirus-covid-19/issue-brief/covid-19-cases-and-deaths-by-race-ethnicity-current-data-and-changes-over-time.

Temel, J. S., J. A. Greer, A. Muzikansky, E. R. Gallagher, S. Admane, V. A. Jackson, C. M. Dahlin, C. G. Blindeman, J. Jacobsen, W. F. Pirl, J. A. Billings, and T. J. Lynch. 2010. "Early Palliative Care for Patients with Metastatic Non–Small-Cell Lung Cancer." *New England Journal of Medicine* 363(8): 733–42.

Tikkanen, R., K. Fields, R. D. Williams II, and M. K. Abrams. 2020. "Mental Health Conditions and Substance Use: Comparing US Needs and Treatment Capacity with Those in Other High-Income Countries." The Commonwealth Fund. Published May 21. http://doi.org/10.26099/09ht-rj07.

US Substance Abuse and Mental Health Services Administration (SAMHSA). 2021. *Key Substance Use and Mental Health*

Indicators in the United States: Results from the 2020 National Survey on Drug Use and Health. Published October 5. http://samhsa.gov/data/sites/default/files/reports/rpt35325/NSDUHFFRPDFWHTMLFiles2020/2020NSDUHFFR1PDFW102121.pdf.

Vahratian, A., S. J. Blumberg, E. P. Terlizzi, and J. S. Schiller. 2021. "Symptoms of Anxiety or Depressive Disorder and Use of Mental Health Care Among Adults During the COVID-19 Pandemic—United States, August 2020–February 2021." *Morbidity and Mortality Weekly Report* 70(13): 490–94. http://dx.doi.org/10.15585/mmwr.mm7013e2.

CHAPTER 8

Improving Coordination and Management Along the Continuum of Care

Success is the sum of small efforts, repeated day in and day out.
Robert Collier, *Riches Within Your Reach*

I FIRST MET Mike when he was being transferred out of the intensive care unit where he had a prolonged stay for an infection and complications from a rare cancer. He was a kind man with a highly complex medical history of surgeries, hospital stays, blood transfusions, and much more. Despite his heavy burden of medical problems, he had a lightheartedness to him that always made me smile. He would joke with me that I needed a second computer system just to keep track of his history and extensive list of medications.

Mike enjoyed spending time with his family. He thought it was destiny that his wife was a nurse. "Thankfully, I married Patty," he told me. "She keeps all my health affairs in line. I don't think I could have afforded her if I had to hire her."

And Patty sure was Mike's lifeline. With his cancer, heart failure, anemia, diabetes, and other medical issues often interacting with one another, she was the one who made sure his conditions were managed properly. Patty had been through the medical system many times, both professionally and with Mike. She understood its strengths—such as critical care—and she also knew its weaknesses—such as providers communicating between one level of care and another.

One evening, Patty called to alert me that Mike was admitted emergently to his local hospital after passing out at a restaurant. He was confused and minimally conscious for the first 24 hours while he was at the hospital. Patty was upset because she saw Mike getting worse. His blood sugars were skyrocketing, and the local hospital was administering a medication regimen without speaking to her. Patty felt frustrated and unheard. I called and spoke to the physician in charge of his case, and we decided to transfer Mike.

When he arrived the next day, I met him and his wife at the hospital. In the 36 hours before I saw him, most of his medications had been either stopped, switched to other meds, or had their dosages changed. Transfer records were sparse, and not all the notes from Mike's hospital stay were transferred with him. My team called to get his full record, and we were told the notes were not complete and would be available for viewing when they were completed.

Patty brought his medication bottles from home when they arrived. Sorting through them, I asked her how he had a prescription for a steroid among the mass of amber vials. Apparently, he was given that when he was released from the rehabilitation facility last month. Now he was being given even higher dosages through his intravenous line.

Wait, what? Mike had a significant history of steroid psychosis on a recent hospitalization and was found to be very sensitive even to low dosages. His sugars were out of control on the steroid, and we had to come up with an alternative regimen for him.

"You are right." Patty sighed as she slumped into her chair, exhausted. "I forgot about that. I should have known." She began crying.

But should she have known? Perhaps Mike's care providers could have built a stronger safety net around Mike to ensure that this type of thing would not happen. Maybe we could have communicated with his rehab facility more clearly and told them not to administer the medication. Perhaps we should have reviewed his rehab discharge medications immediately. Maybe we could have gotten him in to see us quickly after discharge.

Mike clearly would have benefited from a more end-to-end care coordination.

IDENTIFYING AREAS OF OPPORTUNITY

In 2012, the *Journal of the American Medical Association* (*JAMA*) published a seminal study by Donald Berwick, MD, and Andrew Hackbarth titled "Eliminating Waste in US Healthcare." The study identified six domains of waste in the US healthcare system and then quantified how much wasteful spending occurred in those six domains during one year alone. In that study, they found that approximately 34 percent of US healthcare spending could be categorized as waste (Berwick and Hackbarth 2012). Seven years later, *JAMA* published a follow-up study that quantified how much wasteful spending occurred in those six domains from 2012 through 2018. That study found that substantial waste was still occurring, with approximately one in four dollars of US healthcare spending being categorized as waste (Shrank, Rogstad, and Parekh 2019).

The following are the six domains of waste in the study:

1. Failure of care delivery
2. Failure of care coordination
3. Overtreatment or low-value care
4. Pricing failure
5. Fraud and abuse
6. Administrative complexity

While all these domains of waste are important, in the scope of this chapter I am addressing failures and opportunities in how we manage the continuum of care in a value-based system, so I will focus on the first three. To begin, let's explore how these domains are defined:

- **Failure of care delivery.** When we in the healthcare system do not adopt widely accepted best-care processes—such as preventive care and patient safety practices—or execute them well, clinical outcomes suffer while patients endure needless injury and illness. Evidence-guided care is key here. Often, when a provider deviates from evidence-guided care, it is not because they have found a method or process that only they know. Typically, deviations from evidence-guided care result in suboptimal outcomes and higher costs. This relates to the mantra I have repeated in this book: *resilient and effective models of care delivery make the* right *thing to do for the patient the* easy *thing to do for the provider.*

- **Failure of care coordination.** This wasteful spending occurs either because people in our populations are falling through the cracks due to a failure to identify them and connect them with a coordinator, or because we provide them with fragmented care. Failure to deliver coordinated care often results in readmissions, duplicate testing, chronic health complications, and decreased physical and/or cognitive functioning. Navigating the complex health system can be a daunting task. Effective care coordination is particularly vital to the health and functioning of people living with chronic illnesses.

- **Overtreatment or low-value care.** Overtreatment and the delivery of low-value care are the hallmarks of our old fee-for-service mindset in the healthcare system. This wasteful spending comes from ignoring accepted science and the wishes of the beneficiaries in our populations. It includes prescribing medications and performing surgeries that do not improve people's health status or quality of life. It also includes failure to understand and adhere to patient wishes for advanced illness care.

The *JAMA* researchers estimated the following ranges of average annual cost of waste in these three domains: failure of care coordination, $27.2 billion to $78.2 billion; failure of care delivery, $102.4 billion to $165.7 billion; and overtreatment or low-value care, $75.7 billion to $101.2 billion. This results in an estimated annual total cost of $203.5 billion to $345.1 billion wasted in care that lacks benefit to the patient.

Resilient and effective models of care delivery make the right thing to do for the patient the easy thing to do for the provider.

The researchers also projected that annual savings from interventions that address the continuum of care in these three domains have the potential to reduce wasteful spending by $86.8 billion to $163.9 billion. That's a big shared-savings incentive for organizations engaged in value-based care.

ENSURING CARE THROUGHOUT THE CONTINUUM

You will remember a version of exhibit 8.1's continuum-of-care model from chapter 3, when I introduced some of the social driver disparities in the continuum of care. In this variation I am showing the challenges and opportunities along the way. Again, the continuum of care starts with getting the people in our populations on board with a primary care professional.

Primary care is at the top of the list of the World Health Organization's (WHO's) eight actionable priorities in continuity of care, based on published evidence of what works:

1. Continuity with a primary care professional
2. Collaborative planning of care and shared decision-making
3. Case management for people with complex needs

4. Colocated services or a single point of access
5. Transitional or intermediate care
6. Comprehensive care along the entire pathway
7. Technology to support continuity and care coordination
8. Building workforce capability (WHO 2018)

In my practice, focusing on the continuity of care, I strongly agree that all these elements are vital parts of addressing the care continuum. To make this list more comprehensive, I propose a ninth priority: medication therapy management. As most doctors will tell

---

Exhibit 8.1. Opportunities Along the Continuum of Care

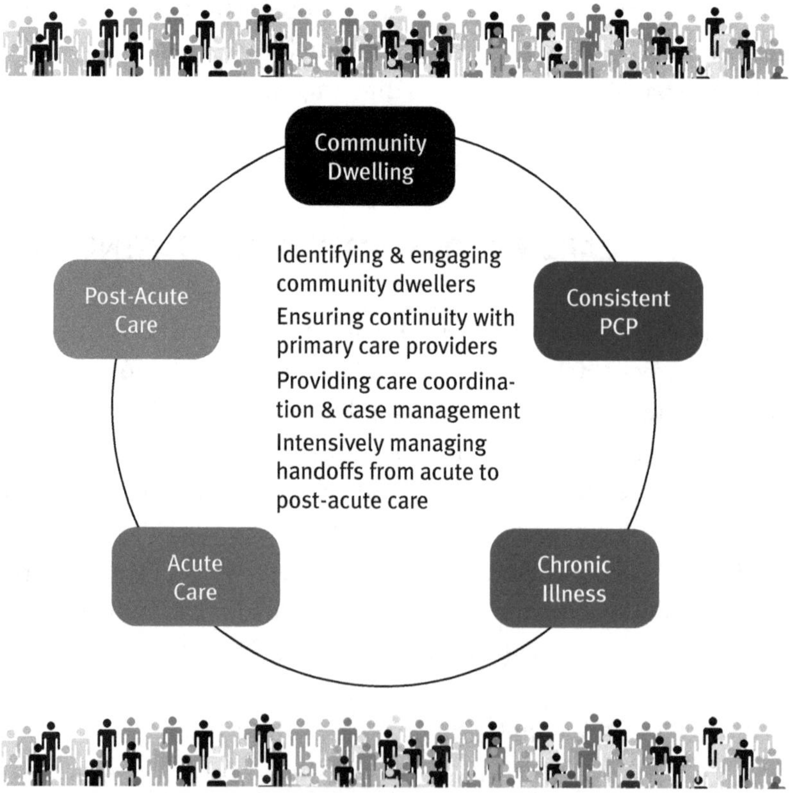

Community Dwelling

Identifying & engaging community dwellers

Ensuring continuity with primary care providers

Providing care coordination & case management

Intensively managing handoffs from acute to post-acute care

Post-Acute Care

Consistent PCP

Acute Care

Chronic Illness

you, if something is going to go terribly wrong in coordinating care between one site and another, it will often be related to medications in transitions. I will explore that shortly.

OPPORTUNITIES IN CARE DELIVERY AND CARE COORDINATION

Throughout this book so far, I have emphasized elements of the opportunities in care delivery and coordination, especially in reducing unnecessary emergency department (ED) visits and admissions. However, far more is involved in coordinating care for a specific population, especially when single or multiple chronic conditions are involved, as is often the case.

First, as discussed in prior chapters, the evidence suggests that care is best coordinated from a primary care professional's office. Studies show that when people have consistent contact with their primary care provider, they show up less in the ED and are admitted to the hospital with less frequency. This makes sense, because when we keep this high-touch relationship, we are giving patients a different access point to the healthcare system. This also gives them access to preventive interventions that help keep them out of unnecessary and more intensive modes of care. We are not doing this with the old fee-for-service mindset of getting as many office visits with them as possible; we are striving to avoid exacerbation and an eventual need for higher-cost modes of healthcare delivery.

Consistent and watchful primary care for populations leads into the second WHO priority of collaborative care planning and shared decision-making. Care in the American health system can be complex. When I see my palliative care patients, I like to ask them an informal poll question: "How many medical visits do you have this week?" I have been astonished to learn that it is not unusual for a patient to have two, three, or more healthcare visits in a week. I have even been told by some patients that I am the third visit of that day! That is a lot of time, a lot of rides back and forth to provider offices, a lot of time in waiting rooms, and most concerning of all, a lot of opinions about how best to manage care.

All this activity can be dizzying to even the most seasoned healthcare professional. Think for a moment about how confusing it could be for a patient to attend all these visits, hear the different opinions, synthesize the data, pull out the yellow pill from their pillbox and add in the blue pill on certain days of the week, only to be told that the generic manufacturer changed on the medication and now both pills are white. It is a wonder that more patients do not end up in the ED with exacerbations of chronic conditions.

In chapter 7 I spoke about patient-centric goals of care. It is important to understand what a patient and their family wish to get out of their care. While many physicians are adept at these conversations, care coordinators are highly focused on patient goals of care. If a patient tells us that they want to be managed in the home, we should try to accommodate that request. Patient-centric goals often center around comfort and independence.

MANAGING COMMUNITY WELLNESS TAKES . . . A COMMUNITY

Typically, care coordination is happening among the primary provider and care managers, who can be nurses or other trained professionals such as pharmacists, social workers, or behavioral health providers. These care-team members are experts at handling the labyrinth that is the medical system and navigating a patient properly through it. They use data often supplied by an ACO or other value-based care organization to attain insight into patient needs and how the existing system can help meet them. Many emerging technologies assist with monitoring patients in their home environment and may augment traditional information to a care coordinator.

Someone who provides care management typically begins with asking patients questions such as the following:

- What is important to you?
- What would you like to result from this condition?
- I understand that your condition has been poorly controlled; what would it take for us to get this better controlled for you?

Generally, a care manager will be able to handle members of a population with a wide range of chronic illnesses, although there are some models in which a care manager might cover a single illness. We see that in some cases, as in patients with severe heart failure. In my palliative care clinic in the cancer center, we have care managers who are dedicated specifically to cancer.

As I have reiterated several times in this book, comprehensive care management is typically performed out of a primary care office. Take the example of a cancer care specialist who is managing the case for one of our patients. We need that specialization to properly manage that patient, but often an event will emerge with the patient that is beyond something cancer care managers regularly see. They may not be adept at managing other co-occurring chronic illnesses, such as diabetes, heart failure, COPD, and other conditions that are outside their specialty. For this reason and others, I tend to prefer care coordination that comes out of the primary care office and think that is the most effective.

TRANSITIONAL CARE: A KEY TO QUALITY OUTCOMES AND LOWER COST

When case management is necessary for people with complex needs, a keen focus on providing quality transitional care is required. A transition point in healthcare is when someone moves from one level of care to another. This can be seen when someone goes from an outpatient setting to an acute inpatient setting or when a hospitalized patient is sent to a skilled nursing facility.

Transitional care is often an inflection point, where things might go either very well or very poorly. Transitional times can be rocky and are common areas for failure. Medications are duplicated or stopped; patients don't receive adequate follow-up; someone along the continuum didn't understand what they were or, more importantly, were *not* supposed to do, all because we didn't make the right thing to do the easy thing to do.

In chapter 4, I summarized a few case studies from the Centers for Medicare and Medicaid Services (CMS) that can be found on its Innovation Models website. They provide examples of programs from ACOs that have improved beneficiary outcomes and resulted in reduced costs. The case study of University of California San Francisco Health is an outstanding example that involves transitions in care and the emphasis on serving patients where they live.

University of California San Francisco Health, whose ACO serves nearly 10,000 beneficiaries in the San Francisco metropolitan area, created its Care at Home program in 2016. The program serves medically complex and homebound beneficiaries by conducting home visits that, in addition to serving patients' clinical needs, also address social drivers and environmental issues that affect them. The Care at Home process starts with identifying patients in need of such a program through referral by providers in inpatient and ambulatory settings and through self-referral. After identification, a physician or nurse practitioner assesses patient needs and environmental factors during an initial visit. If the patient is eligible and consents to be included in the program, they are enrolled and then assigned a primary care provider, who provides care in the patient's home, usually once a month.

In 2018, program leaders compared outcomes of patients enrolled in the program with those who were not, finding that the program participants experienced nearly 70 percent fewer admissions, 65 percent fewer ED visits, and approximately 70 percent fewer observation stays. In addition, a 2019 study found a 95 percent satisfaction rate among those enrolled in the program (CMS 2020).

This example of ensuring adequate care in the community setting is still the exception rather than the rule. There are many points along the care continuum where things fall through the cracks for our beneficiaries.

In writing this chapter on the continuum of care, I interviewed Dr. Catherine Pantik. Dr. Pantik has more than 20 years of experience in transplant science as a practice leader and as a nurse practitioner in acute and post-acute care for kidney transplant recipients. She was also an assistant professor at the Loewenberg College of Nursing at the University of Memphis for more than five years. Pantik is a doctor of nursing practice (DNP) and an advanced practice registered nurse (APRN). DNPs are at the highest level of nursing practice. They specialize in improving patient outcomes and translating research into practice. APRNs have met advanced educational and clinical practice requirements and often provide services in community-based settings.

Dr. Pantik's perspective is valuable for this chapter because she oversees, researches, and teaches in one of the most challenging environments for ensuring the continuum of care—management of kidney transplant recipients. These patients can live long and productive lives after transplant, but successfully achieving that quality outcome depends on adherence to medication and care management plans. This is true for many chronic diseases where there is a handoff from surgery to home, but transplant recipients provide a quintessential example. And it begins with the first handoff—from the transplant center back to the community with the referring nephrologist and the primary care provider.

Many times, even with something as vital as a transplant patient, you don't necessarily get a real handoff. The provider might get an email or a package in their inbox that says, "This is your patient. We're sending them back to you. They had a transplant on this date." So that's a critical piece we're working on—creating a protocol for handoffs between the transplant centers back to the referring nephrologist with the important pieces of information that they absolutely need to know about the surgical procedure itself. What are the key clinical indicators that you must know in order to manage that patient going forward?

Dr. Pantik says that the process of handing off the patient and ensuring the patient knows what to do needs to start much farther back in the patient's plan of care:

This shouldn't start that late in the game. It should be an ongoing conversation that begins when that patient is referred pre-transplant and through their workup and getting them on the transplant list. But it generally doesn't happen that way. It's piecemeal, and the quality of how they communicate varies from center to center. So we try to focus on how we create effective handoffs, and educate the patient too, because the patient has to be engaged, so that they know when they're supposed to be seen again.

She recalls meeting a particular patient in a focus group. By protocol, the transplant center typically sees patients once a year after they've been handed back to the referring nephrologist. This patient claimed she never knew that and she had never been back. Dr. Pantik says, "If she didn't know that and wasn't calling to make these appointments, why wasn't the transplant center or even the general nephrologist ensuring that she was being followed? Why weren't they saying, 'Hey, have you been back for your annual visit with the transplant team?'"

KEEPING CARE IN THE FAMILY

In our population-health and community-wellness activities, these care coordination and case management practices are where we start to involve families and informal caregivers. This is a growing trend that we can take advantage of to help ensure a healthy continuum of care in our communities.

According to a research report by the American Association for Retired Persons and the National Alliance for Caregiving (2020), 53 million US adults were unpaid family caregivers in 2020—way up from 43.5 million when a similar study was conducted just five years earlier in 2015. That means that in 2020, one in five Americans was a caregiver! Nearly a quarter of them (24 percent) were providing care for multiple people, and half of them were caregiving for an older parent.

Often, care coordinators and case managers have better connections with families and caregivers than do other members of the care team. A lot of initial care coordination is done via telephone. In addition to questions about health status, other questions may come up, such as "Who helps you out at home?" Not only may the patient tell you who that is, but that caretaker might also be sitting right next to them during the call. This connection provides "coaches" to those at-home so they know whom to contact in the healthcare system and how to contact them regularly if they need assistance.

Why is it so important to connect with the family caregivers? So many times, we see that the caregivers are our eyes and ears within the home. If you have a family member with multiple chronic conditions, the family has to realize what the individual needs. The family needs to change their dietary lifestyle in certain ways to support that family member. They need to be aware that the patient must be able to make it to their appointments. From a budgetary standpoint, family members often need to try to figure out how they can support the patient so they can afford to continue taking their medications.

Some readers may now be asking the question, "Doesn't Medicare cover these services in the home?" Well, the short answer is no. Medicare can provide some help with home nursing a few times per week. In certain circumstances a home health aide can be deployed as well. But Medicare does not pay for someone to come and live in your house if you have 24-hour care needs.

Making that liaison with the person in the home or the caregiver, especially in the setting of advanced illness, is key. In that setting, it is not unusual that patients are too sick, too lethargic—too anything—to be able to manage themselves. What we need in that home is someone who understands the plan of care and can say, "I've had this conversation with my doctor or with her care manager. Therefore, I'm able to carry this plan forth and call the home care liaison if I need help." It is always worthwhile to have a plan clearly set forth and then a plan B, just in case.

COLOCATING SERVICES

Colocating services is one great way to facilitate smooth navigation through the continuum, but that is not always easy or possible. When I was working at Cooper University Health Care in Camden, New Jersey, they colocated services very well. One of the first places that I worked in Cooper was what we call the medical mall in Voorhees, New Jersey. Located within one building, we had a surgery center, an infusion center, primary care, cardiology, pulmonology, oncology, and more. The center also housed general surgeons, a laboratory, and imaging. Patients appreciated the convenience of it all. The facility even added a lunch area there, and it worked exceptionally well.

These colocations of services provide opportunities for other types of community and social services to be integrated in these areas as well. Dr. Pantik addressed this challenge in our interview. "Even though there are so many services available to people in so many cities, there is often not a singular location where a patient can go for comprehensive services that include social services," she said. "One thing we rely on with social workers is to augment our ability to direct patients to different community service organizations that are available to them. It is difficult to bring those community services together."

While an increasing number of electronic health records (EHRs) now link to community-based organizations, many proprietary platforms still do not communicate well with one another. As we touched on in chapter 6, lack of interoperability in EHRs and healthcare information technology as a whole has long been a challenge, but in recent years, value-based care and the coronavirus pandemic have both been drivers in tackling some of these challenges. One area in which this has been helpful is in the WHO's seventh actionable priority: technology to support continuity and care coordination.

EMPLOYING TECHNOLOGY IN THE CONTINUUM OF CARE

One area in which technology is being used successfully to support continuity and care coordination is evidence-based clinical care pathways. Clinical care pathways are used as a method of managing care of the individual based on evidence-based clinical practice guidelines. The goal of employing these care pathways is to improve care quality, reduce unnecessary clinical practice variation, and ensure effective stewardship of healthcare resources (Chawla et al. 2016).

These clinical care pathways work best when they can be seamlessly integrated into provider workflows at the point of care to augment their practices. In 2018, the University of Chicago Medical Center (UCMC)—the main healthcare institution of the University of Chicago, which serves Chicagoland and northwest Indiana—established its EHR-integrated clinical pathways (E-ICP) program. This clinical pathway program is part of its systemwide high-reliability effort to "promote effective translation of evidence into clinical practice to promote high-value care" (Bartlett et al. 2023, 261).

Patients who are enrolled in clinical care pathways are managed through their EHRs within a pathway platform on which stakeholders (pathway owners and physicians) collaborate throughout the pathway process. The provider delivering care at the point of service is prompted during the visit to adhere to care delivery that is consistent with existing medical evidence. This helps eliminate unexplained deviations in clinical practice.

The E-ICPs were instituted as various clinical conditions and diseases were identified as priorities in a five-phase process with specific timelines. At the time the E-ICP program began, UCMC leadership had no way of knowing that less than two years after its launch this system would be profoundly tested by one of the worst pandemics in modern history.

In a 2022 study, UCMC authors explained how the program helped them meet demands for "rapid information dissemination, resource allocation, and data reporting" created by the pandemic (Bartlett et al. 2022). In March 2020 it became evident that with all the constantly changing federal, state, and city guidance, the E-ICP development process needed to be kicked into high gear. Exhibit 8.2 compares the new COVID-era phases and timelines to the original phases and timelines.

At the outset of the pandemic, 21 pathways were developed and launched in the first 14 days. In all, UCMC developed 45 clinical care pathways that were specific to COVID-19. The study found that some of the major effects of using E-ICPs for COVID-19 included

- expediting the COVID-19 isolation process and supporting resource stewardship,
- driving an optimal COVID-19 testing strategy, and
- enhancing patient triage and internal and external reporting.

The authors concluded that E-ICPs "provide a flexible and unified mechanism to meet the evolving demands of the COVID-19 pandemic" and added that they continue to be a valuable tool in managing COVID-19 (Bartlett et al. 2023, 267).

For the purposes of this book, another part of that final conclusion in the study is noteworthy: "Lessons learned may be generalizable to

Exhibit 8.2. E-ICP Implementation Timelines

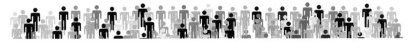

Pre–COVID	During COVID
1. Initiate: 1–2 weeks 2. Plan: 1–2 weeks 3. Design: 2–4 weeks (depending on stakeholder availability) 4. Implement: 2–4 weeks (depending on complexity of requirements and IT changes) 5. Sustain, Improve & Spread: Regular check-ins, formal 30-, 60-, and 90-day assessments	1. Initiate and Plan: 1 day 2. Design: 1 day 3. Implement: 1–5 days 4. Sustain, Improve & Spread: Daily

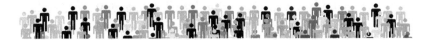

Source: Data from Bartlett et al. (2023).

other urgent and nonurgent clinical conditions." In the next chapter we will explore more about how clinical care pathways can be incorporated into a platform for population health and value-based care.

MANAGING POPULATIONS IN THE ACUTE AND POST-ACUTE SETTINGS: BUILDING A SOUND NETWORK

Retention of a population within a well-defined network of providers is key to successful management. It can be difficult for patients or the primary care delivery team to maintain adequate oversight of the care that is delivered. If our goal is to provide end-to-end care of the individual in order to ensure quality outcomes, it is imperative that we have the ability to work closely with the physicians and other providers who are managing the population that needs acute care.

When we consider our network of high-value providers, we consider those who are interested in whole-person care and maintaining high-quality outcomes. We communicate with providers within our network regularly to make sure they all are aware of our goals and can help to provide such care. While there are times when it makes sense for our beneficiaries to seek care outside the network, we strive to maintain a comprehensive network that is convenient for our populations.

Acute-care providers in a high-value accountable care network are expected to deliver care that is evidence-based and efficient. Communication is essential for optimal care. That communication should be with patients and caregivers, primary care physicians, other specialists, and any post-acute care services. The best hospital teams that are supporting value-based care explore and follow patient wishes for care and connect with outpatient providers where appropriate for what we call the "warm handoff."

Acute-care providers also must ensure that patients have adequate access to care upon discharge and must refer to home-based services where feasible. All patients should be referred to follow-up in a timely manner, usually within seven days. Sometimes that follow-up can be with a primary care physician or with the specialist who saw them in the hospital. As I mentioned previously, discharge medications are frequently an area that needs attention, and a primary care physician usually has comprehensive insight into medication management.

When an individual requires post-acute care in an inpatient setting such as a rehabilitation facility, it is important for an ACO to have relationships with area providers. These relationships should provide the opportunity for the patient to get the services they need in a timely manner and communicate a comprehensive care plan for the longitudinal care of the individual.

DVACO manages the post-acute care cases that are considered to be outliers. We can estimate a length of rehabilitation stay based on a diagnosis and other factors and evaluate beneficiaries who stay beyond that expectation. Is there something we can do to facilitate getting the person home? Is equipment needed? Home nursing? Medications?

ADDRESSING SOCIAL ISOLATION AS A SOURCE OF HEALTHCARE UTILIZATION

Social isolation is a significant driver of healthcare costs and utilization in an elderly population. When individuals are isolated and have no one to care for them, they may end up in the ED for a host of reasons. Some of these include that they are hungry and don't have someone to cook a meal for them, or they need someone to help them get in and out of bed, or they don't remember to take their medications and experience an exacerbation in their chronic condition that puts them in the hospital.

People experiencing social isolation have a higher risk of heart disease, stroke, depression, and anxiety. In fact, a study published by the American Psychological Association demonstrated that social isolation and loneliness were associated with slower gait and decreased ability to carry out the activities of daily living (Shankar et al. 2017). Actual or even perceived social isolation has been found to increase the risk of early mortality (Holt-Lunstad et al. 2015; National Academies of Science, Engineering, and Medicine 2020).

In cases of significant social isolation, those who manage population health must step in with people and innovative technologies to help. Sometimes this type of help may mean home health aides or community health workers. Community health workers may be specifically trained for such interventions to help isolated individuals. But how do we build this workforce capability when we are losing so many in the healthcare professions? This situation is often when innovative technology comes in to help ensure that individuals are safe, taking their medications, and eating properly.

HEALTHCARE WORKFORCE CAPACITY REMAINS STRESSED

The COVID-19 pandemic has truly highlighted many of the short-falls and stress points of the American health system. Even in a set-ting with waning numbers of cases, healthcare workforces remain stretched and stressed to the maximum. As I write this book, hiring levels in healthcare are rising, and the jobs outlook is brighter in the healthcare industry than in many others. That is the short-term view. In the context of 10,000 people becoming seniors each day, it is significantly unlikely that we will be able to meet the needs of this population. That means we must analyze the need and balance that against our mission to be good stewards of our resources, which include our workforce, where there are signs of huge impending shortages.

The following are two sample analyses:

Nursing shortages. The Bureau of Labor Statistics (BLS) report "Employment Projections 2021–2031" estimates that the registered nursing (RN) workforce will grow from 3.1 million in 2021 to 3.3 million in 2031. That's an increase of 6 percent, or 195,400 RNs. Unfortunately, the same analysis also projects that there will be 203,200 openings for RNs in *each year* from 2021 through 2031. Why? Well, our workforce is aging right along with the rest of the population. The pandemic was particularly difficult for RNs, so nurse retirements and exits from the workforce are factored into those calculations. And this is just RNs. The BLS also estimates there will be a need for approximately 30,200 new advanced-practice RNs every year through 2031 (BLS 2022).

Physician shortages. A report released by the Association of American Medical Colleges (AAMC) projects a shortage of between 37,800 and 124,000 physicians in the 15 years between

2019 and 2034. This includes shortages of between 17,800 and 48,000 primary care physicians and between 21,000 and 77,100 non–primary care physicians. The researchers make an interesting point based on our newfound awareness from the pandemic about disparities in care among minorities, rural community dwellers, and people without insurance, as I outlined in chapter 3. "If underserved populations had healthcare use patterns like populations with fewer access barriers, demand would rise such that the nation would be short by about 102,400 (13%) to 180,400 (22%) physicians relative to the current supply" (AAMC 2021, viii).

Action must be taken immediately to reverse these trends, considering the years of education it takes for physicians and nurses to be adequately trained to enter the workforce. Meeting these challenges will mean reimagining not only the workforce but also the entire technology platform for providing value in population health and community wellness. What activities can be automated? What can be done by a different level of training? Are we using a team-based approach to manage our populations? In the next chapter we will explore how that new platform of population health might look.

REFERENCES

American Association of Retired Persons and National Alliance for Caregiving. 2020. *Caregiving in the United States.* Published May 14. http://doi.org/10.26419/ppi.00103.001.

Association of American Medical Colleges (AAMC). 2021. *The Complexities of Physician Supply and Demand: Projections from 2019 to 2034.* Published June. https://www.aamc.org/media/54681/download.

Bartlett, A. H., S. Makhni, S. Ruokis, M. K. Selling, L. Hall, C. A. Umscheid, and C. Kao. 2023. "Use of Clinical Pathways Integrated into the Electronic Health Record to Address the Coronavirus Disease 2019 (COVID-19) Pandemic." *Infection Control & Hospital Epidemiology* 44(2): 260–67. http://doi.org/10.1017/ice.2022.64.

Berwick, D. M., and A. D. Hackbarth. 2012. "Eliminating Waste in US Health Care." *Journal of the American Medical Association* 307(14): 1513–16. http://doi:10.1001/jama.2012.362.

Centers for Medicare and Medicaid Services (CMS). 2020. "Providing Primary Care to Homebound Patients: UCSF Health's Care at Home Program." Published July 15. https://innovation.cms.gov/media/document/aco-casestudy-ucsf.

Chawla, A., K. Westrich, S. Matter, A. Kaltenboeck, and R. Dubois. 2016. "Care Pathways in US Healthcare Settings: Current Successes and Limitations, and Future Challenges." *American Journal of Managed Care* 22(1): 53–62. http://pubmed.ncbi.nlm.nih.gov/26799125.

Holt-Lunstad, J., T. B. Smith, M. Baker, T. Harris, and D. Stephenson. 2015. "Loneliness and Social Isolation as Risk Factors for Mortality: A Meta-Analytic Review." *Perspectives on Psychological Science* 10 (2): 227–237. https://doi.org/10.1177/1745691614568352

National Academies of Sciences, Engineering, and Medicine. 2020. *Social Isolation and Loneliness in Older Adults: Opportunities for the Health Care System.* Washington, DC: The National Academies Press. https://doi.org/10.17226/25663.

Shankar, A., A. McMunn, P. Demakakos, M. Hamer, and A. Steptoe. 2017. "Social Isolation and Loneliness: Prospective Associations with Functional Status in Older Adults." *Health Psychology* 36(2): 179.

Shrank, W. H., T. L. Rogstad, and N. Parekh. 2019. "Waste in the US Healthcare System: Estimated Costs and Potential for Savings." *Journal of the American Medical Association* 322(15): 1501–9. http://jamanetwork.com/journals/jama/fullarticle/2752664.

US Bureau of Labor Statistics (BLS). 2022. "Occupational Outlook Handbook, Registered Nurses." Updated September 8. http://bls.gov/ooh/healthcare/registered-nurses.htm.

World Health Organization (WHO). 2018. *Continuity and Coordination of Care: A Practice Brief to Support Implementation of the WHO Framework on Integrated People-Centered Health Services.* Published November 7. http://who.int/publications/i/item/9789241514033.

Building Platforms for Population Health

Be a yardstick of quality. Some people aren't used to an environment
where excellence is expected.
Steve Jobs

I ALWAYS FOUND it important to keep up on my clinical skills. Since I completed my residency, I knew that being a doctor was something I enjoyed, found rewarding, and am good at doing. Throughout my years of creating systems for managing providers, palliative care, or population health, I still maintained the importance of a steady clinical presence and being out there in front of patients.

In one particularly memorable clinical session, I saw a lovely 67-year-old retired office worker named Martha. Martha was smart and savvy, and she knew the health system all too well. I always smiled when I saw her name on my list for the day because she had a beautiful Jamaican accent that made all of her sentences come out like a song.

Martha knew the health system because she had been through it multiple times in the previous year for chemotherapy and complications stemming from the same. Unfortunately, now Martha was having difficulty recovering in her activities of daily living, likely from a recent hospitalization because of COVID-related pneumonia. Luckily, her cancer was reasonably well controlled.

I saw her the day before Labor Day weekend as my last patient of the day. She was in a wheelchair but was self-propelling quite well. Her mental capacity was excellent. As with many palliative care visits, we started by reviewing her symptoms and schedule of pain medications, followed closely by a conversation about her activities. We then began to review her goals.

"Fall is coming, and it's my favorite time of year," she told me. "I just want to be independent in the house so I can take care of myself and my two cats. I haven't recovered my strength from that last hospitalization. Can you set me up with some therapy in my home, even for a little?"

Now there was a request that I could fill. "Of course," I said. "Did they offer you therapy when you were discharged from the hospital?"

"They did, but I didn't think I would need it. My daughter was going to stay with me, but her husband is sick, so she has to be with him now."

"You got it, Martha," I said. "Can you wait about five minutes while I get the request in order for your therapy?"

I stepped out of the examination room and went back to our social worker to ask what we needed to get some therapy set up in Martha's home. Martha did not need home nursing care, just some strength and balance training to help her regain her independence. Our social worker that day was a very seasoned woman who was covering for our regular team member. She asked that I put the order in the electronic health record (EHR), and she would figure out what needed to be done.

Uh-oh. Now I got a pit in my stomach. How would I do that? I tried typing in "physical therapy," and it did not yield results for home options. I entered "home care," and there was no option for therapy. I tried entering the name of an agency we often used, and it did not come up. I tried a few different variations of home therapy, all without success. By now, the practice nurse and the social worker were starting to sense my frustration and came over to bail me out.

Between the three of us, we were befuddled. They both tried to help me. After a few futile attempts from the three of us, I decided to "phone a friend" and ask another doc in the division. Unfortunately, she had already left for the long weekend and was not available. The nurse and social worker both offered a bevy of what seemed like viable suggestions to enter a simple order for home physical therapy. None of it worked. All of this was while both of them were on the phone trying to find an agency that would accept the referral, all to no avail.

I looked up at the nurse and social worker and said, "Seven advanced degrees between the three of us and we can't figure out how to get home physical therapy services set up." I looked down at my watch, and we were more than 35 minutes in by now. I told Martha that she should just go home with the transport team, and someone would have to call her on Tuesday. I hoped she was able to stay home until then.

As I walked back to the provider room to toil over how to get these services for Martha, it struck me that if I had wanted to send her to the emergency department (ED), it would have taken me less than two minutes.

Now that is a system that is not making the right thing to do the easy thing.

FOUNDATIONS IN CARE COORDINATION

When I think about creating an infrastructure to support population health, the first part we need is a solid care coordination foundation to help people like Martha. As we discussed in chapter 8, care coordination is a team generally composed of nurses, but it can also include pharmacists, integrated behavioral health providers, and medical assistants. Sometimes these teams may be led by nurse practitioners or physicians in addition to the primary care provider. These professionals are dedicated to intensive, one-to-one interactions with patients and to the use of innovative technologies to identify problems and communicate with individuals in need.

Not every patient in a defined population needs care coordination. Some will need services for a short time, such as those who had a recent hospitalization or ED visit. Other individuals will need long-term help because they have a host of challenges related to chronic disease and social drivers of health, which we discussed in chapter 3. Most patients in an accountable care organization (ACO) or associated with a population health team have no immediate need for a care coordinator. These folks may just need someone on standby in case there is a change in their health status.

Recall that in population health, we focus on being good stewards of financial resources in healthcare. That concept includes being good stewards of care coordination resources. For example, care coordination services delivered by a nurse, pharmacist, or other provider involve human capital, information technology (IT) and connectivity to an EHR, space, leadership structure, and more. Without thoughtful application of the service, one can easily envision how costs get quickly out of control.

One of the first issues to approach in utilizing care coordination appropriately is the ratio of care coordinators to a population. Undoubtedly, care coordination ratios vary depending on the population's size and demographics. For instance, a Medicare population requires a more intensive level of attention than a primarily younger and healthier population found in a commercial insurance program.

As I mentioned in chapter 6, figuring out how best to position care coordination requires a close look at your population, parsing out which patients will benefit from the service. Care coordinators engage with patients in order to help to improve outcomes, navigate them through the system, decrease duplication, perform medication reconciliation, and deliver education. One frequently used method to identify those in need is through understanding a population's characteristics. Often populations can be segmented into low-risk, rising-risk, inappropriate utilization or documentation, or high-risk and high-utilization (see exhibit 9.1).

Exhibit 9.1. Care Coordination Categories

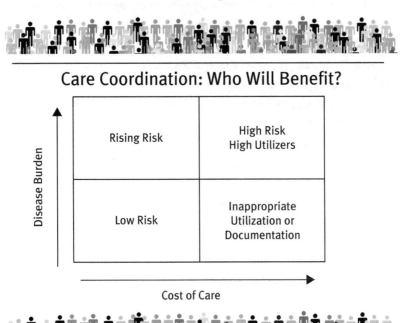

Care Coordination: Who Will Benefit?

Rising Risk	High Risk High Utilizers
Low Risk	Inappropriate Utilization or Documentation

(vertical axis: Disease Burden; horizontal axis: Cost of Care)

While each of these categories requires a different management strategy and carries worth in and of itself, the greatest return on investment is in proactive management of those who are high-risk high utilizers and rising-risk individuals. Preventing one admission in our data not only saves the health system several thousand dollars but also allows a patient the opportunity to remain at home, independent, and in control of their care.

Aneesh Chopra (see chapter 6)—CEO of CareJourney and the first Chief Technology Officer of the United States—says that one of the most important things we can do in population health is to identify the population members who need us most. These are people whom we often miss. He cites what he calls his "operating manual" for reliably delivering on the promise of better quality at a lower cost:

Step one in the operating manual is to keep a list of individuals to call or monitor alongside those you have prepared for when they scheduled to come in to see you. Part of that operating manual involves what computational judgments need to be made, because you won't manually build that list. You might take advantage of all of the computation that's available. So step 2 of the operating manual is to organize the information you have about each of the folks in your panel so that you can formulate a priority list of them to monitor. It is just as important to reach out to individuals to bring them in for more regular care because more primary care delivered to the patients who need it most should translate into fewer emergency room visits and hospitalizations.

PROVIDER MANAGEMENT

As discussed throughout this book, value-based care is a different way to practice in driving better outcomes. Instead of focusing only on the people who are in front of you, you have to figure out who is not in front of you but should be. Who is suffering from chronic conditions but is not coming in to see you? Remember, in population health, finding those "missing persons" is much more about the infinite game of providing the best health outcomes at the lowest cost to the healthcare system.

Still, you must also think about who is coming in today. As a provider organization, you may need to have a morning huddle with your staff and physicians. Typically, morning huddles address questions such as the following:

- What are the needs of the people who are coming in today?
- Do we have all the records for anyone who has had care delivery outside the system?
- Do we understand their social needs?

- Do we have transportation for those who require it to get to us?
- Do we have availability for sick-patient visits today?

Managing a population well is the goal of value-based care, and the morning huddle is an important part of that. The outcome of the morning huddle sounds something like this: "Dr. Angelo, you have six diabetics coming in today, and two of them were uncontrolled when their last labs were checked. The staff will enter orders for these folks for a recheck, and if you agree, please sign the orders when the patient sees you." This is a great way to help keep the focus on the quality of care delivery as well.

QUALITY DASHBOARDS

Integral to managing a practice well in the value-based care arena is the use of analytics to understand, globally, how well your providers are doing in terms of the quality of care. Quality performance is often measured by adherence to industry standards for preventive care such as cancer screenings or vaccination. For individuals with certain conditions, such as hypertension or diabetes, our analytic dashboards tell us whether we are managing these individuals appropriately with good resultant blood pressure or blood sugar control. As I have mentioned many times in this book, quality outcomes are truly key to value-based care performance.

It follows, therefore, that your ability to perform in value-based care is directly related to your ability to measure performance in all attributed patients across multiple important domains within your network. Measuring performance across a cadre of providers helps you understand performance gaps and the positive and negative outliers. Typically, quality performance is quantified in a performance dashboard. That dashboard can be customized per doctor, practice, or other grouping such as region or specialty.

Performance dashboards typically keep information in a single location, where providers and practice leaders can view key performance measures across a provider's entire population. These dashboards will show performance rates compared to benchmarks and are often color-coded red, yellow, or green for an easy view of goal achievement. Quality dashboards will often contain items such as preventive care delivery (mammograms, colonoscopies, and vaccinations), utilization (primary care and specialist visits), and acute care (ED, hospitalizations, and readmissions). As an organization matures in its journey to value-based care, these dashboards include information about average cost of care compared to benchmarks as well.

Transparency is key in helping providers achieve top performance. Most providers want to be top performers and will strive to attain better results based on understanding their performance in relation to that of other providers within the network. Few things are more motivating than showing a doctor that he or she falls in the bottom quartile of the network.

Health system leaders can also use key-performance-indicator dashboards to understand the need for resource allocation to various pockets of the region. For instance, if two practices in a neighborhood are the ones with poorest compliance with retinal exams in diabetics, perhaps additional ophthalmology support in that region is appropriate. Perhaps handheld retinal cameras could be deployed to the primary care practices to help to save a diabetic person's sight.

ELECTRONIC HEALTH RECORDS AND INFORMATICS

The clinical team needs to have the clearest picture possible of the patient's story. This is the job of the EHR, which has evolved greatly over time. The earliest versions of an electronic medical record essentially provided a place for physicians to type their notes and collate them under a patient's name. If you needed a piece of information from that record, you had to know which date you documented it so you could open up the right note.

The EHRs of today have evolved greatly and now often contain a longitudinal view of the patient's care with running problem lists and medication lists. A longitudinal record is a single complete patient record that combines data from all four pillars of population insight—provider-reported data, patient-generated data, health information exchange data, and medical claims data—to provide a complete picture of the patient's story. Social and family histories, as well as health maintenance records documenting preventive health measures, are maintained across multiple specialties. The EHR now can even gather information from multiple sites as well.

The increasing capabilities—and complexity—of the EHR have given rise to the field of clinical informatics. A clinical informaticist is someone with a clinical background who is specially trained to work with data and various IT structures to improve performance, workflow, and management of electronic resources (Silverman et al. 2019). These folks help physicians and other providers deliver care with a focus on quality and performance.

We engage our informatics partners to help in customizing the EHR interface so that providers can focus on delivery of good care and the EHR can prompt the provider if a particular need is seen. This helps our doctors know who needs additional attention or who, for instance, needs an update on their advance-care plan or an evaluation for a risk of falls.

We talk a lot about decreasing cost of care and increasing patient adherence to medications for our beneficiaries. When it comes to adherence to medications, a good informaticist will set up a system whereby prescriptions for chronic medications will default to 90 days. So for people who are on blood pressure medication, when the provider is ready to order a medication, the EHR will default to 90 days to try to make the right thing to do the easy thing to do.

Some organizations are using the EHR for even further evidence-driven practice. These care pathways can prompt a physician to ask certain questions or consider certain medications based on the patient's presentation. With the meteoric rise of artificial intelligence (AI) and its use in healthcare, I predict we will see a major shift toward AI-driven pathways in the coming years. This highlights the skyrocketing importance of a high-performing informatics team and innovative technologies that augment our knowledge of and communication with patients.

HEALTH INFORMATION TECHNOLOGY: THE *WHO* AND *WHERE* OF PATIENT CARE

IT platforms need to understand who and where patients are at any given moment. It may sound simplistic, but it not always clear who the attributed provider is for a given patient. Medicare may indicate one provider for a patient, even though that provider may not have seen that patient after they moved to a different state three months ago. Perhaps a doctor has a new patient on her list whom a commercial payer has erroneously attributed to another physician. Maybe the patient didn't change their provider with their payer, so the provider of record is delayed.

Once we have a handle on the *who*, it is time to focus on the *where*. Are the patients home? Are they in a nursing home? Are they in a rehab facility? Are they in a hospital? It is important that we use platforms to understand where those patients are along the continuum of care at any moment. IT systems may contain an important element called admission discharge and transfer (ADT) feeds. We take that information into account to help us understand, for example, whether a patient was admitted to the hospital last night after being sent to the ED.

ATTENTION TO THE FRAMEWORK FOR POST-ACUTE CARE

Population health management also requires a focus on post-acute care, which generally consists of a tight network of preferred providers. Post-acute care providers include skilled nursing and rehabilitation facilities, home health agencies, hospice providers, and now outpatient rehabilitation therapy providers. The post-acute care team should have visibility into where your patients are at any given moment and understand what the expectations are for the patients.

At DVACO, we use a tool that helps us understand expected length of stay for people in post-acute care. We then manage those who are outliers from our expectations. An example of outlier management could include rehab placement for a patient who was hospitalized with heart failure. Often the initial recommendation is some degree of home nursing plus physical therapy as appropriate. If the patient doesn't have the capabilities or resources to do physical therapy in the home, they may end up in a skilled-nursing facility. While there, the patient will receive rehabilitation services. Our technology helps us understand the expected number of days for which that patient will be confined to the facility, based on their condition and a number of other factors.

If the expectation is that somebody should be in a rehab facility for 10 days but they are there for 15, our team reaches out to understand why this is happening. What are the barriers to progression that may benefit from an intervention? If these barriers are long-term concerns, how do we address this to help keep the patient well-managed upon discharge? I refer to this as a system of accountability.

Most value-based care organizations maintain a tightly managed preferred-provider network. Inclusion on the preferred-provider list requires a high level of quality performance and evidence-based practice. Often, preferred networks are populated by the providers who achieve the best quality and patient experience scores along with ensuring the lowest costs. These are the facilities that are willing to partner with us in order to deliver a better product.

ACCOUNTABILITY FOR QUALITY ON THE CARE TEAM

As part of a comprehensive population health platform, it is imperative to have a knowledgeable quality team leader. This leader needs to know all the measures for which the care team is being held accountable and the ongoing trends in achieving those quality targets. Quality leaders must understand performance targets and where performance sits at any given moment. Your quality leader and their team should also be adept at understanding the complex regulations that come from CMS and commercial programs.

In chapter 4, where we examined ACOs, we learned about organizations achieving shared savings for decreasing the cost of care compared to expected costs. Above all, value-based care is not about cost cutting as much as it is about quality performance. Quality performance, as measured by attainment of various targets across a network, will often determine the percentage of shared savings you will earn for your financial performance. Some programs have a quality "gate"—a single number for performance—while others have a "ladder" whereby higher quality performance results in an incrementally higher shared savings percentage for your organization.

Undoubtedly, cost cutting in the absence of quality focus will decrease the amount of provided care. Unrestrained cost cutting is never the ultimate goal in population health. High-quality outcomes and patient experience of care are the keystones to success. In value-based care, if your quality fails to meet a minimum threshold, you will likely receive zero reimbursement from that shared savings.

The Healthcare Effectiveness Data and Information Set (HEDIS) is a tool used by many health plans and quality departments to measure quality performance across several domains. I introduced this concept in chapter 5. Medicare Star Ratings are used for Medicare Advantage programs and are the culmination of quality performance in patient experience surveys as well as several HEDIS measures. In 2023, Consumer Assessment of Healthcare Providers and Systems (CAHPS) scores are expected to determine more than half of an organization's star rating.

PATIENT EXPERIENCE

In your quality department, you want to ensure that you have visibility into the patient experience as measured by the CAHPS survey tools. There are Hospital CAHPS (for hospital care), Clinician and Group CAHPS (for primary care and specialty office care), and other measures of patient experience. These surveys are standardized and statistically honed instruments that measure patients' experience of care with providers and other team members in each of these settings.

For many reasons, it is important for organizations to focus on the patient's experience of care. Patients who have a better experience with their healthcare providers will listen to what their providers say, are more likely to adhere to their orders and care plans, and are more likely to have better health outcomes (Doyle, Lennox, and Bell 2013; Trzeciak et al. 2016). If the providers do not connect well with their patients, they will probably never see that patient again, and the patient will probably not follow through on orders from that provider.

I have always been a strong proponent of the patient experience. When I was at Cooper University Health Care, I worked with a group on patient experience. We researched the correlation between patient experience, cost of care, and Medicare Star Ratings for hospitals. In a study of more than 3,000 hospitals around the country, a better hospital patient experience, measured by Medicare hospital star ratings, was associated with lower Medicare spending per beneficiary. On average, hospitals with the highest patient experience star rating spent 5.6 percent less than hospitals with the lowest star rating (Trzeciak et al. 2017).

PAYER CONTRACTING IN THE POPULATION HEALTH PLATFORM

When ACOs initially began to surface, they were focused on CMS programs such as the Pioneer ACO or the Medicare Shared Savings Program as the main vehicle for value-based care. More recently, healthcare leaders have recognized the opportunity for performance and savings through additional value-based care programs such as commercial insurance, Medicare Advantage, or Medicaid managed care products. That has driven the need for a payer contracting team with expertise in value-based care.

As such, many ACOs now have a payer-contracting leader dedicated to their population health platform. These are people who are experts at managing relationships with payers. Those relationships are important because they become the bedrock for our relationships with patients and providers in a value-based program. In many settings, an organization may have a typical fee-for-service agreement with a payer. They may also have a value-based agreement on top of that.

High-quality value-based care performance requires a solid network of providers with whom you are working. In a population health infrastructure, it is important to have a network development leader who can communicate with providers and be the "face" of value-based care for affiliated doctors. Network development leaders will recruit new providers while helping to manage performance among existing participants.

MANAGING THE NECESSARY PRACTICE TRANSFORMATION

Value-based care is transformational—no two ways about it. If it is not, you are not doing it right. Everyone in your organization is taking on responsibility for the health of a population, driving quality health outcomes for patients while also becoming conscientious stewards of the organization's resources. This is far more than we ever asked of our workforce in the fee-for-service world.

In chapter 3, I introduced the Quintuple Aim and the importance of keeping these factors in mind as we strive toward transforming our organizations toward value-based care (see exhibit 3.3 on page 40). Solid performance in community health management means transforming the way everyone practices, from the office staff to the clinicians to the CEO. Given this new paradigm, it is important to provide a framework for the effective delivery of care (see exhibit 9.2) This requires a person or team of people who are focused on what we call practice transformation, which encompasses all of the new things you are asking your people to do that may differ from typical fee-for-service activities.

Solid performance in community health management means transforming the way everyone practices, from the office staff to the clinicians to the CEO.

Practice-transformation functions in population health include a wide array of issues. For example, patient access can be increased through an on-call service that has access to the patient's EHR to help people through their questions or problems. Practices might

Exhibit 9.2. Practice Transformation Framework

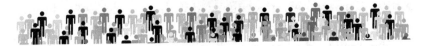

- ☑ Patient Access—during and after office hours, phone access, sick visits
- ☑ Quality Performance—using evidence-based care delivery, performance across a set of care measures, agrees to data transparency
- ☑ Resource Stewardship—organization agrees to focus on cost by using generic drugs where appropriate, managing patients in the home if feasible, preventing avoidable ED visits, and referring to care coordinators
- ☑ Clinical Documentation—organization agrees to properly document the illness burden of all patients
- ☑ Citizenship—practice agrees to meet with ACO team for performance review, and providers agree to conduct educational sessions
- ☑ Regulatory Reporting—practice uses certified EHR, performs annual compliance program, and is able to report on quality

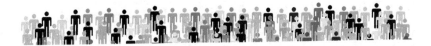

also work on gaining better visibility into quality performance and resource stewardship.

Practice-transformation team members are heavily involved with the practices. They educate the providers and office staff about value-based care initiatives and help them understand components of the system that they need to work on for their programs to succeed. They also will have a deeper understanding of CMS regulations for value-based care participation, and they can have other information that is helpful to practices so that they can ensure compliance with any regulations required for successful participation in the program.

PHYSICIAN AND PROVIDER LEADERSHIP

The best way to get provider buy-in is to have providers help create the infrastructure for population health. After all, doctors and nurses who are facing patients every day will often have the best perspective on what will work and what will require additional effort to achieve success. Changes that are embedded within a practice tend to be the most beneficial to patients.

The medical director for value-based care plays a key role in practice transformation efforts for providers. This medical director is generally a physician who understands the needs of the providers and the patients. They work with the network director, quality leader, analytics team members, and other practice leaders across their attributed practices to understand successes and challenges to performance. These doctors give an ACO the provider and patient perspective while helping develop programs for success.

DIVING IN

It is widely accepted that you won't learn how to swim by dipping your toes in the water. Similarly, you won't succeed in population health or value-based care without a clear-cut commitment to the process that starts with the right leadership. The extensive list of infrastructure elements needed to create a functional population health program makes it sound nearly unattainable. I won't sugarcoat it: it's hard. But the rewards can be great both in quality outcomes and financial performance.

I am only scratching the surface in this chapter. Some health systems may have many of the pieces of a population health team already in place. Getting all of these pieces to harmonize together is truly transformational and creates a new paradigm of care. Our work here will never be finished.

You can have a lucrative engagement. You can decrease the cost of care and share in some of those savings. And you can create a win–win situation whereby patients get the right amount of care without duplication or wasteful services. Best of all, patients will experience care that is managed and navigated properly while receiving high-quality outcomes.

Given the high cost and mediocre quality of the US health system as it exists now, we are faced with two options: we can manage the cost and quality on our own or wait for someone else to step in and manage it for us. I prefer to be on the leading edge of that change.

In the final chapter, I will explore some of the challenges and changes on the horizon that have the potential to make population health, community wellness, and value-based care a more pervasive reality in the US healthcare system.

REFERENCES

Doyle, C., L. Lennox, and D. Bell. 2013. "A Systematic Review of Evidence on the Links Between Patient Experience and Clinical Safety and Effectiveness." *BMJ Open* 3 (1): e001570.

Silverman, H. D., E. B. Steen, J. N. Carpenito, C. J. Ondrula, J. J. Williamson, and D. B. Fridsma. 2019. "Domains, Tasks, and Knowledge for Clinical Informatics Subspecialty

Practice: Results of a Practice Analysis." *Journal of the American Medical Informatics Association* 26(7): 586–93.

Trzeciak, S., J. P. Gaughan, J. Bosire, and A. J. Mazzarelli. 2016. "Association Between Medicare Summary Star Ratings for Patient Experience and Clinical Outcomes in US Hospitals." *Journal of Patient Experience* 3(1): 6–9.

Trzeciak S., J. P. Gaughan, J. Bosire, M. Angelo, A. S. Holzberg, and A. J. Mazzarelli. 2017. "Association Between Medicare Star Ratings for Patient Experience and Medicare Spending per Beneficiary for US Hospitals." *Journal of Patient Experience* 4(1): 17–21. http://doi.org/10.1177/2374373516685938.

CHAPTER 10

Into the Future of Value-Based Care

*Seeing modern health care from the other side, I can say that it is
clearly not set up for the patient. It is frequently a poor arrangement
for doctors as well, but that does not mitigate how little the system
accounts for the patient's best interest. Just when you are at your
weakest and least able to make all the phone calls, traverse the maze
of insurance, and plead for health-care referrals is that one time
when you have to—your life may depend on it.*
Ross Donaldson, *The Lassa Ward: One Man's Fight Against
One of the World's Deadliest Diseases*

SOME PROVIDER ORGANIZATIONS will go to extraordinary
lengths to make sure people do not fall through the cracks. Tackling healthcare's hurdles for this population calls for an aggressive
strategy; typical brick-and-mortar primary care practices need a
more transformative approach.

AbsoluteCare is an example of an organization that, according to
their motto, goes "Beyond Medicine." They provide for the medical,
behavioral, and social needs of member populations in Louisiana,
Maryland, Ohio, and Pennsylvania. AbsoluteCare accepts risk contracts with payers, taking over the healthcare management needs of
the top 1 to 2 percent of the costliest patients. They often take on
the most challenging patients in terms of chronic illness burden and
social drivers of health, and they manage them well.

"Whether we are going out into the community or seeing members in our comprehensive care center, we attend to *all* health needs," says Greg Foti, MD, AbsoluteCare's chief medical and transformation officer. "That's what it means to go *beyond* medicine" (Foti and Raman 2023).

The AbsoluteCare team of physicians, nurses, social workers, case managers, pharmacists, and others employ unique methods to help their members adhere to their medical regimens. If patients miss appointments, AbsoluteCare sends out a transport van to do a wellness check and may bring them in for their chronic illness check-in. Sometimes the team will have to do some exploring in the community to locate members through family or friends, especially members experiencing housing challenges. Often, staff will bring members into the AbsoluteCare comprehensive care center, give them their medications and a sandwich and a place to be monitored for the day, and then let them go at nighttime to try to maximize their living situation and keep them out of the hospital.

"Our value-based healthcare model is unique," says Anoop Raman, MD, chief medical officer of complex care for Absolute-Care, "and it is always evolving to meet the needs of our members, our teammates, and our health plans. Put simply, it is quality over quantity" (Foti and Raman 2023).

Patients feel well cared for in this model and appreciate that their providers want to see them thrive. When patients do well, AbsoluteCare does well.

RETURN ON INVESTMENT

The defining quality of a major disruptive innovation in any industry boils down to return on investment (ROI). Attending to population health and community wellness to provide value is a noble endeavor, but unless any pursuit, however virtuous, provides value that attracts investment, it will be short-lived. The US healthcare system's history is rife with industry-transformation theories that have been derailed by our coziness with the fee-for-service ecosystem, despite its inherent unsustainability.

As with any disruptive innovation that requires hard changes and propels people out of their comfort zone, value-based care has a number of barriers and ongoing detractors. Let me address the ROI in value-based care, which so far have only been hinted at in this book.

The coronavirus pandemic hobbled many industries and businesses around the world. For example, the restaurant industry was drastically scaled back. The pandemic's effect on the US healthcare delivery system also was devastating. One of the few segments of the industry that thrived during the pandemic's height was value-based care.

In a recent research article, global management consulting firm McKinsey & Company reported, "Value-based care is emerging as a distinct healthcare landscape." Researchers noted that "value-based care quadrupled during the pandemic" while "new hospital construction—a proxy for investment in legacy care models—held flat" (Abou-Atme et al. 2022, 1). Exhibit 10.1 shows that value-based care investment grew faster than new hospital construction during the two-year height of the pandemic.

"Providers specializing in value-based care have become attractive to investors because of the distinctive quality of care that they can provide and the investable opportunity they present, with a diversity of risk levels and business models," the authors write, adding that "continued traction in the value-based care market could lead to a valuation of $1 trillion in enterprise value for payers, providers, and investors."

To create the environment for any disruptive innovation in healthcare or any other industry, there must be *compelling factors*, such as a demonstration of the ability to achieve ROI and produce some excitement around that. There must also be *facilitating factors*,

Exhibit 10.1. Value-Based Care Investment Versus Hospital Construction During the Pandemic

Value-based care investment inflows have grown faster than capital expenditures on new hospital construction.

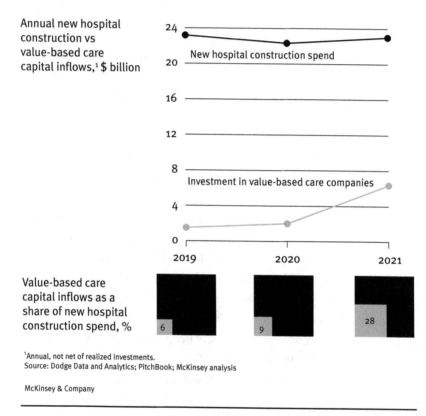

Annual new hospital construction vs value-based care capital inflows,[1] $ billion

New hospital construction spend

Investment in value-based care companies

Value-based care capital inflows as a share of new hospital construction spend, %

[1]Annual, not net of realized investments.
Source: Dodge Data and Analytics; PitchBook; McKinsey analysis

McKinsey & Company

Source: Reprinted with permission from Abou-Atme et al. (2022).

such as technology and interoperability that enable us to achieve what we say we can deliver in population health. See exhibit 10.2 for an in-depth view of the compelling and facilitating factors in value-based care.

Exhibit 10.2. Compelling and Facilitating Factors

Compelling Factors	Facilitating Factors
• A lack of accountability for quality and outcomes in the existing fee-for-service system	• Advancing technology in artificial intelligence and machine learning
• Unsustainable costs in healthcare, especially for the senior and Medicaid populations	• New laws and regulations supporting EHR interoperability
• Consumerism and the desire for better access, experience of care, and patient-driven outcomes	• Strong data and analytics
	• Alternative-payment-model payments for providers to attract participation
• Increased quality reporting and transparency regulation	• New payment agreements between payer organizations that reward quality and efficiency

HEALTH POLICY AND THE FUTURE OF VALUE-BASED CARE

The future of value-based care—and thus, population health and community wellness activities—will be heavily dependent on advancing policy initiatives, especially from the Centers for Medicare and Medicaid Services (CMS). This is not only because of the aging of the population but also because CMS is a bellwether for how commercial payers structure their payment models for healthcare services.

In the realm of value-based care and population health, one of the most active professional organizations is the National Association of ACOs (NAACOS). For this book I interviewed Tony Reed, the current NAACOS board chair, about the organization's priorities in moving value-based care forward. Reed is highly respected in the field of value-based care and has more than 25 years of experience in healthcare, including with Christiana Care, Geisinger Health System, Ascension Health System, and B. Braun Medical, Inc.

NAACOS focuses on major policy initiatives to ensure continuation of programs such as the Advanced Alternative Payment Model bonuses for qualifying participants who take on greater amounts of risk in government programs. This bonus was originated by the Medicare Access and CHIP Reauthorization Act (MACRA) of 2015. Many ACOs feel that this bonus has served as an impetus for provider participation in value-based care.

Mark Angelo: What are NAACO's primary areas of emphasis now?

Tony Reed: One of the key things I want to focus on is: How are we being efficient with the care that we're providing? The aim of the Advanced Alternative Payment Model concept is to incentivize physicians for taking higher levels of risk, and to ensure they are not just walking in blindly, unprepared to go into that risk. The model arrives at a much different result than the proponents of MACRA ever could have envisioned. No one knew how quickly this would catch on and expand. The number of people in ACOs and going to higher levels of risk in the government program show that MACRA was successful in creating the necessary groundwork. Now we must refine that.

Angelo: Do you see that incentive as being meaningful for organizations to support internal initiatives for care coordination, analytics, or other population health infrastructure?

Reed: Yes, in value-based care we do not have all of the mechanisms that have been built out over the years in the fee-for-service structure. There is a great amount of fee-for-service opportunity within value-based care, but many of the elements we are providing and building in value-based care have yet to be reimbursed. Take social determinants of health, for example. Now, we finally have Z codes so we can start billing for those services, establish charges, and put them out there. Even though we established those charges, the government is slow to enact payment for them. Up until that point, we were paying for these services by ourselves, investing in that future, and not having any kind of a reimbursement mechanism to help sustain or start it up.

HOW FAR DO WE HAVE TO GO?

Not all leaders in healthcare are convinced that value-based care will be the thing that finally breaks the US healthcare system's cycle of poor outcomes and runaway costs. David Shulkin, MD, became the ninth US Secretary of Veterans Affairs (VA) under President Trump in 2017. His responsibility included the entire VA delivery system. Shulkin now manages a range of activities from veterans and health policy to working with integrated health systems to working with new companies for innovative care delivery. I asked him whether policy is leading us more toward value-based care and whether he believes that we can jump that chasm soon. Shulkin replied:

> The way you asked the question brings me back to the origins of why I got interested in this. Right when I started training, even as a medical student, I saw a disconnect—that the people involved in delivering and ordering the services had no idea what the cost of that care was. I remember that I almost got thrown out of my residency because I did a study in which I asked the doctors, the nurses, the ward clerks, and the patients how much a test cost—a complete blood count, a chest X-ray, and a CAT scan. When I finished the survey, I found that the ward clerks were the ones who were most accurate. The doctors were the least accurate. When it made the newspapers,

and I published this little study in the *New England Journal of Medicine*, it embarrassed the administration enough that I almost got thrown out of my residency.

I knew at that point that this disconnect was going to lead to the loss of autonomy of the medical profession, because I saw what was happening back when I was training with the rise of managed care. The whole reason for managed care was that doctors and hospitals were not managing the price of care and employers needed a solution. We have been on this path of ignoring the value equation in healthcare for decades. And we are now getting to a point where we are in a race between *can value-based healthcare actually deliver a reduction in the overall spend for value* or *is health policy going to be moving us toward price setting?*

Shulkin stands out among physicians in his desire, early on in his career, to understand the healthcare payment system. In fact, when he first came out of medical training, he did not go straight into a practice or a health system but instead went to work with Blue Cross Blue Shield so he could gain some inside knowledge of the payer world.

This gives him some unique insights into how payers and providers interact. Shulkin says he believes that, so far, the payvider model is not living up to expectations for change in the healthcare industry:

I believe that even in organizations that have both payers and providers, there still has been this wall and silo between them. And I do not see most health systems that have payer organizations acting any differently than any other provider. A true payvider needs to break down the wall between the payer and the provider and operate as a new and unique entity. And I just have not seen that.

There is some interesting work being done in some of the payviders. InterMountain is organizing itself differently to accomplish some of those goals. Kaiser is also a very interesting example that is culturally different than many other payviders. There are some others as well. But many organizations that have developed providers and payers as part of their system have done that as a hedge.

Shulkin contends that health systems have entered their payvider arrangements to diversify revenue streams or protect against competitive forces in the marketplace rather than considering the relationship as fully transformative. Expanding on how to create success in the payvider relationship, Dr. Shulkin states, "We need to redesign the way that healthcare can be delivered. I do believe in the promise of the payvider. I do believe that the financial incentives and the clinical incentives should be aligned together. But I do not see that there are many organizations that are truly doing that today."

Dr. Shulkin also continues to warn of the slowness of implementation of value-based care: "In the past 10 years, I would say it has been increasing in semantics and it is increasing in our presentations and our experimentation. To those like you and me who have run ACOs, it is very real to us, but to a hospital CEO, it still is a minority of the way that they run their business."

OPPORTUNITIES IN VALUE-BASED CARE

Will existing or soon-to-be-implemented value-based payment systems be adequate to facilitate the continued movement toward value-based care? When I consider that question, one novel CMS program that comes to mind is the launch of the ACO Realizing Equity, Access, and Community Health (REACH) model. ACO REACH payment agreements are an example of one of those *facilitating factors* discussed earlier in this chapter. They facilitate a provider's transition into taking on more risk.

As with all accountable care programs, the primary goal of ACO REACH is to manage patients with chronic conditions to improve quality, outcomes, and value in care delivery. The benefits that ACO REACH provides include

- wider use of telehealth,
- waiving the requirement for a three-day inpatient hospital stay before patients can be admitted to a skilled-nursing facility,
- cost-sharing support for copays,
- rewards for successfully managing chronic diseases,
- more generous use of post-acute care home visits, and
- most importantly, advancing health equity in underserved communities.

ACO REACH offers a unique opportunity for managing complex population needs. The REACH model provides an innovative payment approach whereby the ACO can contract with specific hospitals or post-acute delivery sites and create payment opportunities for high performance. In ACO REACH, participant organizations are allowed to create reimbursement structures that support quality and efficiency. Historically, payment structures with provider organizations strictly flowed from health insurance carriers.

ACO REACH participation options include a model centered on primary care or a global capitation model through which the ACO directly pays providers for all services based on an individual's total cost of care. Specialists and acute-care delivery sites get to have some security as a preferred provider, while the ACO can maintain accountability for cost and quality in those sites through payments.

THE CRYSTAL BALL OF CMS

CMS messaging has been clear in that the agency wants 100 percent of Medicare beneficiaries in a value-based arrangement by 2030 (Seshamani, Fowler, and Brooks-LaSure 2022). Those arrangements can be through Medicare Advantage, an ACO, or some other emerging model that focuses on value in the coming years. In the same NAACOS address I highlighted in chapter 2, CMS Administrator Chiquita Brooks LaSure laid out the importance of this issue: "We are charting a new chapter, in which we are laser-focused on health equity, paying for healthcare based on value, and delivering person-centered care that meets the people where they are. We must all work together toward this vision—healthcare that treats the whole person to achieve better health outcomes by advancing equity" (Brooks-LaSure 2022).

Undoubtedly, with the Medicare insolvency crisis looming over the coming years, controlling costs through value-based care is not a movement that CMS regulators or US lawmakers are likely to ignore. We are at a historic point in US healthcare where we can work to control costs in our delivery system, or we can wait for the government or other entity to do that for us.

In addition to the benefits of value-based care to patients and populations described in this book, payers such as CMS favor these arrangements. Sharing the risk of population cost with providers allows CMS to focus on its own budget stability. Consider another thought experiment: Suppose we gave $100 million to an organization that is now in charge of managing a population of 10,000 individuals with high-quality outcomes. Patients should expect good access with a positive experience. Providers inside that organization are incented to manage the population well. The administrative structure should be lean. The acute-care delivery sites are incented to prevent hospital-acquired infections, delays in care, and readmissions. The delivery system wins by doing the right tests and procedures on the right patients. Additionally, the payer organization has some degree of budget certainty.

We are at a historic point in US healthcare where we can work to control costs in our delivery system, or we can wait for the government or other entity to do that for us.

THE RISE OF ALTERNATIVE-DELIVERY
MODELS OF CARE

Retail health clinics, innovative home-based services, and other novel primary care delivery models will play an expanding role in the delivery of care across America in the coming years. Well-resourced, forward-thinking organizations such as CVS, Amazon, UnitedHealthcare, and Walgreens have made major strides in recent years toward being the provider sites that patients identify for their healthcare needs. Patients turn to these organizations for good reason. In each of these models, large companies have decided to move forward from the legacy model of care delivery and create models that focus on cost and patient experience (Anderson 2023).

I heard an interesting lecture recently from a professor from the MIT AgeLab. The professor pointed out some of the differences in generational approaches to healthcare access. The point he made was that generations born after Generation X would be much less likely to access healthcare in the same way it has been accessed for many years. Calling a doctor's office and waiting on hold to make an appointment in four weeks, where you spend the bulk of an afternoon in an office waiting room and exam room for a 15-minute visit with the physician, is not going to be the future of medicine.

Transformed models of care that incorporate telehealth options have increased in popularity, especially since the pandemic. Some employers now offer "telehealth first" programs, in which patients use telehealth initially for medical issues that are not urgent. We have seen the rise of telebehavioral health, gender-based telehealth options, and telehealth for chronic illness management. While the COVID pandemic made telehealth instantaneously possible on a much larger scale than before, ongoing consumer demand will not allow that option to be eliminated.

The increasing presence of wearables that convey information about health will only continue to expand. Individuals can know their heart rate, sleep patterns, and blood oxygenation at any given moment with an affordable watch or ring. Patients with diabetes can collect information on a continuous glucose monitor and transmit it to a provider sitting across the street or across the country to obtain recommendations for insulin management. It is easy to envision that data going to an artificial intelligence or machine-learning algorithm that monitors patients in their homes and produces results on par with even the best physicians.

In the newest models centering on care from primary care providers, where payers and providers collaborate, we will continue to see transformed models dominate. Payvider relationships between primary care service delivery and large payers will continue to engage new healthcare consumers and manage an increasing percentage of the market, such that traditional models of primary care may be challenged. Some innovative primary care models—including AbsoluteCare, as described at the beginning of this chapter, and other models such as Oak Street Health, ChenMed primary care for seniors, One Medical, and Centerwell Primary Care—have already seen remarkable success in this journey.

UNDERSTANDING WHO WILL PAY FOR ALL THIS

In the Preface for this book, I emphasize that we need to do a better job at explaining value-based care to the people in our populations. It is important for patients to know not only that they participate in a value-based care program but also what we are doing for them and why we are doing it. Dr. Shulkin clearly describes this as an opportunity in healthcare where communication is particularly important:

> I think healthcare insurance is the least understood product that a consumer buys. When someone buys a car, they understand the warranty they get from the manufacturer, and then they are offered an extended warranty. When they buy a product that breaks, such as an iPhone, they know they can either get Apple support, or they know where their local store

is. But I do not think people understand the insurance they have, especially the high deductibles they pay when they go to the doctor. They are shocked at what they owe and what the insurance company pays, but they also do not really understand the arrangements there are among the doctors, the hospitals, and the payers.

Dr. Shulkin says that much of the discussion of transparency issues in healthcare has focused on the transparency rule on hospital charges and billing, but he points out that it is not having much of an effect because it is too difficult to interpret. "That is not particularly meaningful," he says. "But the transparency that now needs to happen is creating an understanding of how healthcare is paid for and where the potential solutions are through changing these financial arrangements, such as value-based care. Transparency is going to be helpful in moving this along."

HEADING INTO THE FUTURE WITH BOTH EYES OPEN

To quote Dr. Robert Shmerling (2021), senior faculty editor for Harvard Health Publishing, the US healthcare system is "expensive, complicated, dysfunctional, and broken." There has never been a point in history where so much stress and focus has been on the healthcare system to transform into a more viable model. Remaining within the status quo is prohibitively expensive, in terms of dollars as well as opportunities for better care and outcomes.

Throughout this book, we have explored various challenges and opportunities to better understand how value-based care can address the needs of our communities with real-world solutions that improve care from all aspects. We have examined technology such as innovative analytics and outreach. We have explored the importance of breaking down divisions between payers and providers to finally achieve the goals that our populations need to attain better health.

We have heard from many industry experts who have deployed these programs to achieve success.

Value-based care and the population health approach are disruptive to the status quo. We have our work cut out for us. Certainly, the business of healthcare will continue to cautiously watch the rise of value-based care. During this historic post-COVID time of financial pressures coupled with an aging population and the impending insolvency of the Medicare Trust Fund, we are compelled more than ever to take action, to decrease administrative burdens, and to create a paradigm of transparency and stewardship.

We have the right technology. We have the skill. We must lean in with integrity toward the opportunity to create a system that will be there to serve us when we someday need it most. At that point, we can look up from the stretcher and be proud of what we created, knowing that we, too, will be the beneficiaries.

> *Never doubt that a small group of thoughtful committed citizens can change the world; indeed, it is the only thing that ever has.*
> Margaret Mead, American anthropologist

REFERENCES

Abou-Atme, Z., R. Alterman, G. Khanna, and E. Levine. 2022. "Investing in the New Era of Value-Based Care." McKinsey & Company. Published December 16. http://mckinsey.com/industries/healthcare/our-insights/investing-in-the-new-era-of-value-based-care.

Anderson, M. 2023. "Why CVS and Walgreens Are Targeting Value-Based Care." *Healthcare Brew*. Published March 3. http://healthcare-brew.com/stories/2023/03/03/cvs-walgreens-value-based-care.

Brooks-LaSure, C. 2022. "Opening Plenary." National Association of Accountable Care Organizations Fall Conference. Video, 44:48. http://naacoslive.com/archive/6962.

Foti, G., and A. Raman. Interview with author. April 7, 2023.

Seshamani, M., E. Fowler, and C. Brooks-LaSure. 2022. "Building on the CMS Strategic Vision: Working Together for a Stronger Medicare." *Health Affairs*. Published January 11. http://healthaffairs.org/do/10.1377/forefront.20220110.198444/full.

Shmerling, R. H. 2021. "Is Our Healthcare System Broken?" *Harvard Health Publishing*. Published July 13. http://health.harvard.edu/blog/is-our-healthcare-system-broken-202107132542.

Index

Note: Italicized page locators refer to exhibits.

AAMC. *See* Association of American Medical Colleges (AAMC)

AbsoluteCare, 151–52, 163

ACA. *See* Affordable Care Act (ACA)

Access to healthcare: generational approaches to, 162; US ranking among high-income countries, 8. *See also* Health equity

Accountability: new paradigm of care for population health and, 17; for quality on the care team, 143–44. *See also* Transparency

Accountable care: models of success in, 53–55; what it looks like, 22–23

Accountable care organizations (ACOs), xii, 22–23, 41, 43–55, 59, 84, 116, 118, 136, 145; behavioral population health objectives and, 98; central role of, 55; chronic-illness management and, 38; data-driven decision making for, 51; defining, 46; focus of, xx–xxi, 46; history of, 46–47; home-based palliative care and, 102–3; payer-contracting leaders and, 146; risk continuum and, *48*, 48–49; risk-sharing and, 47; today and tomorrow, 49–51; value-based care and, 18–23; value stories of, 73. *See also* Value-based care

ACO REACH model, 84; benefits of, 160; increase in beneficiaries served by, 49–50; primary goal of, 159–60

ACOs. *See* Accountable care organizations (ACOs)

Activities of daily living: social isolation and impact on, 127

Acute care: delivery, 45; utilization, 38

Acute-care providers: in high-value accountable care networks, 126

Adherence to medications: informaticists' role in, 141

Administrative efficiency: US ranking among high-income countries, 8

Admission discharge and transfer (ADT) feeds: in IT systems, 142

Admissions: preventing avoidable, accountable care and, 53

Advanced Alternative Payment Model bonuses, 156

Advanced-care planning, 23

Affordable Care Act (ACA): accountable care organizations and, 47; population health boosted by, xviii

Age: differences in behavioral health management and, 95–96

Aging population: healthcare workforce stress and needs of, 128; in United States, 12–14, 24

AI. *See* Artificial intelligence (AI)

Alcohol abuse, 89–90

Alda, Alan, xv

Alternative-delivery models of care, rise of, 162–63

Alternative Payment Models (APMs), 47, 84
Altruism: truisms *vs.*, 3–4
Alzheimer's disease: depression and, 92
Amazon, 75, 162
American Association for Retired Persons (AARP), 121
American Psychological Association (APA), 96; social isolation study, 127
Analytics: payvider's role in, 68–69. *See also* Intensive analytics
Anxiety, 91; chronic conditions and, 91–92; social isolation and, 127
APA. *See* American Psychological Association (APA)
APMs. *See* Alternative Payment Models (APMs)
Apollo's Arrow (Christakis), xiii
Apple Health app, 77
Artificial intelligence (AI), 141, 163
Ascension Health System, 156
Association of American Medical Colleges (AAMC): physician shortages report, 128–29
Atrius Health (Massachusetts): Behavioral Health Fellowship, 98–99
Autoimmune diseases: depression and, 92
Autonomy, 6

Bankruptcies: long-term-care facilities and, 13
B. Braun Medical, Inc., 156
Behavioral health: variance in definition of, 94–95
Behavioral healthcare: barriers to, in population health management, 95–96; breaking down the barriers to, 96–99; expanding care beyond, 104; telebehavioral health benefits, 99, *100*
Beneficiaries: Medicare, benefits given through ACO participation, 50–51
Berwick, Donald, 57, 111
Big data, 74–75; as key element in population health, 15, *16*
Billing: medical claims and, 78; transparency issues and, 164

Binge drinking, 90
Black patients: continuum inequities and, 39–40. *See also* Race and ethnicity
Blood-glucose monitors, continuous, 77
BLS. *See* Bureau of Labor Statistics (BLS)
Blue Cross Blue Shield, 158
BRCA testing, 27
Breast cancer screening, 27–28
Brooks-LaSure, Chiquita, 22, 161
Bureau of Labor Statistics (BLS): "Employment Projections 2021-2031" report, 128
Butte, Atul, 71

Call centers: intensive analytics used in, 86–87
Cancer: depression and, 92; outcomes, early stage diagnosis and, 30
Capitation: risk continuum and, *48,* 49
Care: collaborative planning of, 113; retention, importance of, 52; STEEP, six aims or domains of, ix; understanding gaps in, 85. *See also* Accountable care; Care coordination; Continuum of care
Care After Covid (Nundy), xiii
Care coordination, 23, 116; categories in, 136–37, *137*; failure of, defining, 112; failure of, estimated annual cost of, 113; failure of, vignette, 109–11; foundations in, 135–38; frustrating gaps in, 133–35; new paradigm of care for population health and, 17; opportunities in care delivery and, 115–16; population management in acute and post-acute settings and, 125–26; ratio of care coordinators to a population in, 136; resource stewardship and, 136; supporting, technology for, 114; teams in, 135. *See also* Continuum of care
Care coordinators: family caregivers and, 121
Caregiver education, 23
CareJourney, 80, 137
Care management: comprehensive, 117; as key element in population health, *16,* 17

Care managers: role of, 17

Care process: US ranking among high-income countries, 8

Case management: for people with complex needs, 113

Case managers: family caregivers and, 121

Centers for Disease Control and Prevention (CDC), 29; on health inequities, 30; report on mental illness and COVID-19 pandemic, 93–94

Centers for Medicare & Medicaid Services (CMS), 22, 148, 155, 160, 161; Innovation Models website, 53, 98, 118; Medicare fee-for-service beneficiaries' goal set by, 50; Medicare Physician Group Practice Demonstration, 47; national health spending projections, 14; risk "glide path" and, 21–22; virtual care reimbursement, 35

Center to Advance Palliative Care (CAPC): Project Equity workgroup of, 39

Centerwell Primary Care, 163

ChenMed primary care, 163

Chopra, Aneesh, 80, 137

Christakis, Nicholas, xiii

Christiana Care, 156

Chronic illness/disease: coexistence of emotional and physical conditions and, 91–92; mental health disorders and, 93; palliative care and management of, *103,* 103–4; population health focus and, 15; prevalence and management of, 38; telehealth and management of, 162

Churchill, Winston, 43

Citizenship: in practice transformation framework, *147*

Clinical care pathways, 123

Clinical documentation: in practice transformation framework, *147*

Clinical informaticists: role of, 141

Clinical informatics, 141

Clinical interventions: as key element in population health, 15, *16*

Clinician and Group CAHPS, 145

Close, Glenn, 89

CMS. *See* Centers for Medicare & Medicaid Services (CMS)

Collaboration: payer-provider, creating a path for, 59

Collaborative planning of care, 113

Collier, Robert, 109

Colocations of services, 122–23

Commercial insurance, 145

Commonwealth Fund, 8

Community health management: solid performance in, 146–47

Community health workers, 127

Community wellness, 9, 24, 27–41, 96; addressing social factors impacting health, importance of, 32–35, *33;* advancing, psychologists and role in, 97–98; community involvement in, 116–17; continuum inequities and, 39–41; continuum of care and, 36–39, *37;* COVID-19 pandemic issues and, 35–36; equity in population health and, 29–30; examining the obstacles to health, 30–31; family caregivers and, 120–22; models of success in accountable care and, 53–55; Quintuple Aim and, *40,* 40–41; return on investment and, 152. *See also* Continuum of care; Health equity; Population health; Social drivers of health

Compelling factors: in value-based care, 153, 154, *155*

Comprehensive care, 114

Confidentiality. *See* Patient confidentiality

Consumer Assessment of Healthcare Providers and Systems (CAHPS) scores, 144

Continuum management: new paradigm of care for population health and, 17

Continuum of care: addressing, 36–39; closing gaps in, 41; colocations of services and, 122–23; disparities in, 36, *37;* employing technology in, 123–25; family caregivers and,

120–22; gaps in, example of, 109–10; importance of care retention, 52; improving coordination and management along, 109–29; inequities tied to, 39–40; opportunities along, 113–15, *114*; population management in acute and post-acute settings and, 125–26; resilient, creating, 69; supporting, technology for, 114; transitional care and, 118. *See also* Care coordination

Cooper University Health Care, Camden, NJ, x, xvii, 122, 145

Cost cutting: value-based care and role of, 144

Cost of healthcare: evidence-based practice and decrease in, 19; failure in addressing health equity and, 31; by provider, visual analytics and story behind, 82, *83*; Quintuple Aim and, 40, *40*. *See also* Reimbursement

COVID-19 pandemic, x, xiii, 6; E-ICP program at University of Chicago Medical Center and, 124, *125*; healthcare workforce stress and, 128; health disparities within communities of color and, 31; independent providers and, 5; mental health issues related to, 93; social drivers of health and, 35–36; telehealth options and, 162; value-based care during, 153; value-based care investment *vs.* hospital construction during, 153, *154*

Crossing the Quality Chasm (IOM), ix, x

CVS, 162

Dashboards, 16

Data: ACO, 51; converting from raw to cooked, 81–84; health information exchange, 75, *76*, 77, 141; medical claims, 75, *76*, 78, 141; patient-generated, 75, *76*, 77, 141; payvider's role in, 68–69; provider-reported, 75, *76*, 76–77, 141; value added with, 74–75. *See also* Intensive analytics

Data analytics, 75

Data observations: as key element in population health, 15, *16*

Deductibles, 164

Delaware Valley Accountable Care Organization (DVACO), xi, xii, 57, 58, 60, 62, 68; home-based palliative care and, 102–3; post-acute care management at, 127, 143

Deloitte, 31

Depression, 91; chronic conditions and, 91–92; social isolation and, 127

Diabetes: depression and, 92

Diaper sales: aging population and, 12–13

Difficult news, handling in stages, 72

Discrimination, 30

Disease management: palliative care in, 103–4, *103*. *See also* Chronic illness/disease

Disparities in healthcare: physician shortages and, 129

Disruptive innovation: return on investment and, 153

Doctor-patient relationship: value of population health approach in, 15

Donaldson, Ross, 151

Downside risk: risk continuum and, *48, 49*

Drug abuse, 91, 93

Duplicate testing: failure of care coordination and, 112

DVACO. *See* Delaware Valley Accountable Care Organization (DVACO)

DVACO/Humana payvider relationship: history behind, 62; using as a model, 64

Economic stability: as a social driver of health, *33, 34*

Education access and quality: as a social driver of health, *33, 34*

Education programs: payvider relationships and, 66

Effective care, ix

Efficient care, ix

EHR-integrated clinical pathways (E-ICP) program: at University of Chicago Medical Center, 123–24, *125*

EHRs. *See* Electronic health records
(EHRs)
Elderly population: addressing social
isolation in, 127
Electronic health records (EHRs), 87,
136; informatics and, 140–42; lack of
interoperability in, 122–23;
provider-reported data in, 76, *76*
"Eliminating Waste in US Healthcare"
(Berwick & Hackbarth), 111
Emergency department (ED), 34; acute
care utilization and, 38; continuum
inequities and use of, 39; reducing
unnecessary visits/admissions, 115
"Employment Projections 2021-2031"
report (BLS), 128
Epilepsy: depression and, 92
Equitable care, ix
Equitable care delivery and outcomes:
new paradigm of care for population
health and, 17
Equity. *See* Health equity
Ethnic inequality, 29. *See also* Race and
ethnicity
Evidence-guided care: deviations from,
112

Facilitating factors: in value-based care,
153, 154, *155*
Failure of care coordination: defining, 112;
estimated annual cost of, 113
Failure of care delivery, 111; defining, 112;
estimated annual cost of, 113
Family caregivers: connecting with,
120–22
Fee-for-service billing, provider notes
and, 76
Fee-for-service environment: health
information technology use in, *vs.* in
value-based care, 80–81
Fee-for-service model, 6, 18, 41, 46, 47,
59, 153; overtreatment or low-value
care and, 112; risk continuum and,
48, *48*
Finite game: infinite game *vs.,* 19–20
Fitbit tracker, 77
Food deserts, 32

Food insecurity, 28
Foti, Greg, 152
Full-risk programs: risk continuum and,
48, 49
Funding solutions, innovative, 24
Future of value-based care, 151–65; CMS
messaging and, 160–61; health
policy and, 155–57; implementation
challenges and, 159; moving beyond
the status quo, 164–65; opportunities
in, 159–60; return on investment
and, 152–54; rise of alternative-
delivery models of care, 162–63;
transparency issues in payment and,
163–64

Galea, Sandro, x
Geisinger Health System, 156
Gender-based telehealth options, 162
Gender inequality, 29
Gibbins Advisors, 13
Graying of America, 12–14, 24
Gross domestic product: US healthcare
expenditures as percentage of, 8, 14

Hackbarth, Andrew, 111
Handoffs: transplant recipients and, 119,
120; "warm," 126
Harvard Health Publishing, 164
Health: examining obstacles to, 30–31
Health, language, and tech literacy:
disparities in continuum of care
and, *37*
Healthcare: all-consuming work of, xvi;
complicated nature of, xv; playing
the infinite game in, 19–21
Healthcare access. *See* Access to healthcare
Healthcare access and quality: as a social
driver of health, *33, 34*
Healthcare delivery: aging population
and, 14; failure of, 111, 112, 113;
moving beyond paternalistic
approach to, 100–101; opportunities
in care coordination and, 115–16;
picking the right site of service, 45;
rise of alternative-delivery models
of care, 162–63; two scenarios

of, 1–2. *See also* Accountable care organizations (ACOs); Healthcare outcomes; Teams

Healthcare disparities: addressing continuum of care and, 36–39, *37*; COVID-19 pandemic and, 31

Healthcare Effectiveness Data and Information Set (HEDIS), 60, 144

Healthcare improvement movement: three waves in, ix–x

Healthcare industry: graying of America and impact on, 13–14

Healthcare insurance: communication and transparency issues related to, 163–64

Healthcare markets: specific needs of, 61

Healthcare outcomes: best possible, fostering, 15; care retention and, 52; infinite game and focus on, 104; Quintuple Aim and, 40, *40*; social factors contributing to, 24; strong performance on quality and, 85; success in value-based care and, 60; transitional care and, 117–20; US ranking among high-income countries, 8; value-based care and, 80. *See* Value-based care

Healthcare providers: advice for, xxi; care retention and, 52; incentives within salaries for, 4; in independent practices, 4–5; need for payers, 59–61; in payvider arrangements, 66; resilient and effective models of care delivery and doing right by, 112, 113; retention of population within defined network of, 125; shortages of, 128–29; stress of COVID pandemic on, 5; taking on risk, 21–22; use of term in text, xx. *See also* Nurses; Physicians; Primary care providers (PCPs)

Healthcare system: perverse incentives and, 7, 9

Healthcare utilization: social isolation addressed as source of, 127

Health equity, xiii, 24, 161; defining, 29–30; goal of, 30; improved,

Quintuple Aim and, 40, *40*; intensive analytics and issues related to, 73–74; payviders, value-based care, and, 67; in population health, 29–30

Health inequities: COVID-19, mental health issues, and, 94; overcoming, 30

Health information exchange (HIE) data: longitudinal record and, 141; as pillar of population exchange, 75, *76*, 77

Health information technology: in fee-for-service world *vs.* value-based care, 80–81; as the *who* and *where* of patient care, 142

Health policy: future of value-based care and, 155–57

Healthy-eating programs, 17

Healthy People 2030 initiative (HHS), 33

Heart disease: depression and, 91–92; social isolation and, 127

HEDIS. *See* Healthcare Effectiveness Data and Information Set (HEDIS)

HHS. *See* US Department of Health and Human Services (HHS)

High-cost drugs: data analysis of use in ambulatory settings, 82

High-value providers: communicating with, 126

HIV/AIDS: depression and, 92

Holiday, Ryan, 57

Home-based monitoring equipment, 77

Home-based palliative care, 102–3

Home-based services, innovative, 162

Home health agencies, 142

Home health aides, 127

Hospice care, *103*, 104

Hospice providers, 142

Hospital-based care, 45

Hospital CAHPS, 145

Hospital construction: COVID-19 pandemic and value-based investment *vs.*, 153, *154*

How Covid Crashed the System (Angelo & Wohlforth), x

Huddles, 138–39

Humana, xi, xii, 60, 62. *See also* DVACO/
     Humana payvider relationship
Humana/MGMA study on intensive
     analytics, 87, 88
Hypothyroidism: depression and, 92

*If I Understood You, Would I Have This
     Look on My Face?* (Alda), xv
IHI. *See* Institute for Healthcare
     Improvement (IHI)
Incentives: innovative funding solutions
     with, 24; misguided focus of, 6;
     organizational, using alternative
     payment models for, 84; within
     salaries for providers, 4. *See also*
     Perverse incentives
Independent practices, 4–5
Infinite game: focus on outcomes and,
     104; playing, 19–21, 23
Informatics: electronic health records
     and, 140–42
Institute for Healthcare Improvement
     (IHI): Triple Aim, 40
Institute of Medicine (IOM): *Crossing
     the Quality Chasm,* ix, x; *To Err Is
     Human,* ix
Insulin management, 163
Integrated behavioral health providers:
     care coordination and, 135
Intensive analytics, 71–88; as driver
     behind value stories, 72–74; four
     pillars of population insight in,
     75–78, *76*; health inequities and,
     73–74; as key element in population
     health, 16, *16*; organizational
     behavior and use of, 84; patient
     experience improved with, 85–87;
     payvider's role in, 68–69; role of, in
     population health and value-based
     care, 80–81; value-based care and
     momentum toward, 87–88
InterMountain Healthcare, 158
Interoperability: in electronic health
     records, lack of, 122–23; in payvider
     relationships, 69; value-based care
     arrangements and, 87
IOM. *See* Institute of Medicine (IOM)

Jefferson College of Population Health, xi
Jefferson Health, 52, 62
Jobs, Steve, 133
Joint ventures, 63
*Journal of the American Medical
     Association (JAMA),* 111, 113

Kaine, Tim, 80
Kaiser Family Foundation: report on
     COVID-19 pandemic and health
     inequities tied to mental health
     issues, 94
Kaiser Permanente, 158
Keystone ACO: Health Navigator
     Program, 53–54
King, Martin Luther, Jr., 27

Lassa Ward, The (Donaldson), 151
Life expectancy, 41
Loneliness, 91
Longitudinal care, 45
Longitudinal patient records, 140–41
Long-term-care facilities: bankruptcies
     and, 13
Low-value care. *See* Overtreatment or
     low-value care
Lucet (formerly Tridiuum), 85

Machine-learning algorithm, 163
Main Line Health, 62
Managed care, 158
Marginalized populations: vulnerability
     of, 29
McKinsey & Company, 153
McMahon, Cori, 85, 86, 94–95
Mead, Margaret, 165
Medicaid, 18, 79, 145–46
Medical assistants: care coordination
     and, 135
Medical claims data: longitudinal record
     and, 141; as pillar of population
     exchange, 75, *76,* 78
Medical errors: deaths related to, ix
Medical Group Management Asso-
     ciation (MGMA): joint study with
     Humana, on intensive analytics,
     87, 88

Medical groups, large, 4
Medicare, 18, 79, 121, 142; annual
    growth rate in spending and,
    14; beneficiaries, value-based
    arrangements and, 160–61;
    insolvency crisis, 161, 165; Pioneer
    ACO Program, 47; telehealth
    reimbursement, 35
Medicare Access and CHIP
    Reauthorization Act (MACRA)
    of 2015, xviii, 47; Advanced
    Alternative Payment Model bonuses
    and, 156
Medicare Advantage, 62, 79, 145, 161; star
    rating system, 60, 61, 85, 144, 145
Medicare Physician Group Practice
    Demonstration (CMS), 47
Medicare Shared Savings Program
    (MSSP), 47, 49, 57, 58, 145
Medication: access, disparities in
    continuum of care and, *37*; refills,
    80; therapy management, 114
Mental health: chronic illness and impact
    on, 93
Mental healthcare: behavioral healthcare
    and, 94–95; social stigma and, 95–96
Mental illness: COVID-19 pandemic and,
    93; in the United States, 91, 93
MIT AgeLab, 162
Morning huddles: questions to address
    in, 138–39
MSSP. *See* Medicare Shared Savings
    Program (MSSP)
Multiple sclerosis: depression and, 92
Multistate delivery models, 4

National Alliance for Caregiving, 121
National Association of ACOs
    (NAACOS), 49, 73, 155, 156, 161
National Committee for Quality
    Assurance (NCQA): on population
    health management, 23
National health spending: CMS
    projections, 14
National Institute of Mental Health
    (NIMH), 92; on benefits of
    telebehavioral health, 99, *100*

NCQA. *See* National Committee for
    Quality Assurance (NCQA)
Neighborhood and built environment: as
    a social driver of health, *33, 35*
Network development leaders, 146
New England Journal of Medicine, 158
NIMH. *See* National Institute of Mental
    Health (NIMH)
Nundy, Shantanu, xiii
Nurse practitioners, xx
Nurses, 17; care coordination services
    delivered by, 135, 136; population
    health leadership and, 148; shortages
    of, 128

Oak Street Health, 163
Obama, Barack, 80
Obstetrics & Gynecology, 30
Ochsner Health System, 68
OneCare Vermont, 54–55
One Medical, 163
Outlier management, 143
Outpatient rehabilitation therapy
    providers, 142
Overtreatment or low-value care: defining,
    112; estimated annual cost of, 113

Palliation: definition of, 101
Palliative care: in disease management, *103,*
    103–4; expanding care beyond, 104;
    focus of, xviii; home-based, 102–3;
    intersection with population health,
    101–3; shared decision-making and,
    101
Pantik, Catherine, 119, 120, 122
Parkinson's disease: depression and, 92
Patient access: in practice transformation
    framework, *147. See also* Access to
    healthcare
Patient-centered care, ix
Patient-centric goals, 99, 100–101, 104, 116
Patient confidentiality: crucial importance
    of, xxi
Patient data, gathering, 79–80. *See also*
    Data
Patient experience: CAHPS survey
    and visibility into, 144–45; good

performance and, 61; improved,
Quintuple Aim and, 40,
40; intensive analytics and
improvement in, 85–87
Patient-focused goals of care: new
paradigm of care for population
health and, 17
Patient-generated data: longitudinal
record and, 141; as pillar of
population exchange, 75, *76,* 77
Patient Protection and Affordable Care
Act of 2010. *See* Affordable Care Act
(ACA)
Payer contracting: in the population
health platform, 145–46
Payer-provider relationship:
reengineering, xii–xiii
Payers: provider need for, 59–61
Payvider model: evolution of, 61–62;
shortcomings with, 158–59
Payvider relationships: achieving
interoperability in, 69; collaboration
in, 59; evaluating success of, 67–68;
helping financial risk concerns on
both sides, 65–66; risk continuum
and, *48,* 49; types of, 62–64;
value-based care and, 67
Payviders: role of, in data and analytics,
68–69
PCPs. *See* Primary care providers (PCPs)
Performance measurement: quality
dashboards and, 139–40
Performance targets: quality leaders and,
144
Perverse incentives, 1–9; behavioral
economics for physicians, 5–7;
rethinking reimbursement, 8–9;
roaring inefficiencies of American
medical care, 7–8; a tale of two
Saras, 1–3; understanding medical
practices in America, 4–5
Pharmacists, 17; care coordination services
delivered by, 135, 136
Physician assistants, xx
Physicians, 17; autonomy of, 6;
behavioral economics for, 5–7; care
coordination and, 135; population

health leadership and, 148; shortages
of, 128–29; use of term in text, xx
Pioneer ACO Program, 47, 145
Podiatric medications demonstration,
71–72
Population-based payments: risk
continuum and, *48,* 49
Population health, 9, 11–24, 44,
96; advancement of, xviii–xix;
committing to, 148–49; creating
populations from people, 14–15;
equity in, 29–30; family caregivers
and, 120–22; four pillars of
population insight and, 79; health
equity goal in, 29–30; identifying
population members who most need
care in, 137–38; intensive analytics as
ultimate driver of action in, 72–74;
intersection with palliative care,
101–3; keeping pace in, 23–24; key
elements of, 15, *16*; models of success
in accountable care and, 53–55; new
paradigm of care for, 17; payvider
relationships and, 66; physician and
provider leadership for, 148; playing
the infinite game and, 19–21, 23;
practice-transformation functions
in, 147–48; psychologists and role
in, 97–98; resource stewardship
and, 136; return on investment
and, 152; role of analytics in, 80–81;
shared decision-making and,
100–101; taking on risk and, 21–22;
value-based payment models and,
xx, 18. *See also* Community wellness;
Health equity; Resource stewardship
Population health agreement, 18
Population health management: barriers
to behavioral health in, 95–96;
definition of, 23; foundational
aspects of, 23–24; goal of, 23;
post-acute care focus and, 142
Population health platform: payer
contracting in, 145–46
Population insight, four pillars of, 75–76;
health information exchange data,
75, *76,* 77, 141; medical claims data,

75, *76*, 78, 141; patient-generated data, 75, *76*, 77, 141; provider-reported data, 75, *76*, 76–77, 141
Post-acute care, 38–39; attending to framework for, 142–43; comprehensive care plan for, 126–27
Poverty, 30, 34, 36
Practice transformation: framework for, *147*; managing, 146–48
Preferred-provider network: value-based care organizations and, 143
Prescription drug data: podiatric medications demonstration, 71–72
Preventable (Slavitt), xiii
Prevention: population health management and focus on, 24
Preventive medicine, 15
Primary care: focus on, xx
Primary care models: innovative, 162, 163
Primary care physicians: shortages of, 129
Primary care providers (PCPs): care coordination and, 135; chronic-illness management and, 38; comprehensive care management and, 117; continuity with, 113, *114*; continuum of care and, 36–37; lack of access to, 34; reduced ED visits and care coordination with, 115
Provider management: morning huddles and, 138–39
Provider network development: care retention and, 52
Provider-reported data: longitudinal record and, 141; as pillar of population insight, 75, *76*, 76–77
Providers: disparities in continuum of care and bias of, *37*; Quintuple Aim and well-being of, 40, *40*. *See also* Healthcare providers; Primary care providers
Psychologists: population health approach and role of, 97–98
"Psychology's Role in Advancing Population Health" policy (APA), 96–97

Quality: of care delivery, accountable care and, 22–23; "gate," 144; "ladder,"
144; outcomes, transitional care and, 117–20; targets, new paradigm of care for population health and, 17
Quality dashboards, 139–40
Quality on the care team: accountability for, 143–44
Quality performance: in practice transformation framework, *147*; value-based care and, 144
Quintuple Aim, 24, *40, 40–41*, 146

Race and ethnicity: continuum inequities and, 39; COVID-19, mental health issues, and, 94; healthcare disparities and, 30–31
Racial inequality, 29
Raman, Anoop, 152
RBRVS. *See* Resource-based relative value scale (RBRVS)
Readmissions: failure of care coordination and, 112
Reed, Tony, 155, 156–57
Registered nurses (RNs): shortages of, 128
Regulatory reporting: in practice transformation framework, *147*
Rehabilitation facilities, 142, 143
Reimbursement: rethinking, 8–9; risk-sharing relationships and, 63, *63*; transactional care and, 6; for virtual care, 35
Reliance Healthcare: ED care-coordination program, 53
Renaudin, George, 68, 69
Resource-based relative value scale (RBRVS), 6
Resource stewardship, 18, 23, 61, 136; care retention and, 52; cost of care by provider and, 82–84, *83*; healthcare workforce stress and, 128; new paradigm of care for population health and, 17; in practice transformation framework, *147*; prescription cost management and, 72
Retail health clinics, 162
Return on investment (ROI): in value-based care, 152–54

Risk, taking on, 21–22
Risk coding: educating providers in, 66
Risk continuum: accountable care and, *48, 48*–49
Risk-sharing, 18, 47
Risk-sharing relationships, 62–63; financial performance and, 64; types of, 62–63, *63*
Robert Wood Johnson Foundation, 29
Robust analytics: as key element in population health, 16, *16*
ROI. *See* Return on investment (ROI)
"Role of ACOs in Addressing Health Equity, The" (National Association of ACOs), 73

Safe care, ix
Salaries: incentives within, 4
SAMHSA. *See* Substance Abuse and Mental Health Services Administration (SAMHSA)
Sexual orientation, 29
Shared decision-making, 17, 100–101, 113, 115
Shared-savings arrangements: risk continuum and, *48,* 49, *50*; risk-sharing relationships and, 64
Shmerling, Robert, 164
Shulkin, David, 157, 158, 159, 163, 164
Silos: eliminating, 65
Sinclair, Upton, 1
Sinek, Simon, 11, 19
Single-sided risk: risk continuum and, *48,* 49
Skilled nursing facilities (SNFs), 84, 142, 143
Slavitt, Andy, xiii
Smoking-cessation classes, 17
SNFs. *See* Skilled nursing facilities (SNFs)
Social and community context: as a social driver of health, *33,* 35
Social and family histories: longitudinal record and, 141
Social determinants of health: use of term, 31; Z codes and, 157
Social drivers of health, 31, 32–35; COVID-19 pandemic and, 35–36;

definition of, 32; disparities in continuum of care and, *37*; economic stability, *33,* 34; education access and quality, *33,* 34; examples of, 32; five domains of, *33*; healthcare access and quality, *33,* 34; negative, overcoming, 36; neighborhood and built environment, *33,* 35; social and community context, *33,* 35
Social factors: impacting health, importance of addressing, 32–35; that contribute to health outcomes, 24
Social isolation: addressing as source of healthcare utilization, 127
Social workers, 122
STEEEP care: outlined in *Crossing the Quality Chasm,* ix
Stress management sessions, 17
Stroke: depression and, 92; social isolation and, 127
Substance Abuse and Mental Health Services Administration (SAMHSA), 90–91
Substance use disorder, 91
Suicidal ideation: social stigma and, 95
Suicide rate: in the US, 93
Systemic racism: disparities in continuum of care and, *37*

Target, 75
Teams: AbsoluteCare, 152; accountability for quality on the care team, 143–44; within accountable care organizations, 23; in care coordination, 135; chronic-illness management and, 38; new paradigm of care for population health and, 17; payer contracting, 146; post-acute care, 142–43; practice transformation management and, 147–48
Technology: employing in continuum of care, 123–25; social isolation issues and use of, 127. *See also* Artificial intelligence; Electronic health records (EHRs); Telehealth
Telebehavioral health, potential benefits of, 99, *100*

Telehealth: barriers to, 36; reimbursement for, 35; "telehealth first" programs, 162

Thomas Jefferson University system, 52

Timely care, ix

To Err Is Human (IOM), ix

Transitional care, 114; quality outcomes, lower cost, and, 117–20

Transparency: healthcare insurance and, 163–64; top performance and, 140. *See also* Accountability

Transplant recipients: transitional care for, 119–20

Transportation: lack of, 32

Triple Aim (IHI), 40

Trump, Donald, 157

Two-sided risk: payvider relationships and, 65–66; risk continuum and, *48, 49*

Uninsured population, 34

UnitedHealthcare, 162

United States: aging population in, 12–14, 24; prevalence of mental illness in, 91, 93; roaring inefficiencies of medical care in, 7–8; understanding medical practices in, 4–5

University of California San Francisco Health: Care at Home program, 118–19

University of Chicago Medical Center (UCMC): EHR-integrated clinical pathways program at, 123–24, *125*

Upside risk: risk continuum and, *48, 49*

Usage patterns: data analysis of, 81–82

US Census Bureau: aging population estimate, 12

US Department of Health and Human Services (HHS): on aging US population, 12; Healthy People 2030 initiative, 33

Uterine cancer: healthcare disparities and, 31

Value-based care, xx, 29, 51, 55, 164; accountable care organizations and, 18–23; bipartisan support for, 47; chronic-illness management and, 38; committing to, 148–49; definition of, 18; genesis of accountable care and, 46; good outcomes and, 60; health information technology use in, *vs.* in fee-for-service environment, 80–81; identifying areas of opportunity for, 111–13; medical director for, 148; momentum toward intensive analytics and, 87–88; patient engagement and, 79; payer contracting teams and, 146; payviders and the march toward, 67; provider management and, 138–39; quality dashboards and, 139–40; quality performance and, 144; return on investment in, 152–54; role of analytics in, 80–81; shared decision-making and, 100–101; status quo and disruption of, 165; taking on risk and, 21–22; transformational nature of, 146; "warm handoffs" and, 126. *See also* Accountable care organizations (ACOs); Community wellness; Future of value-based care; Health equity

Value-based payment models: population health and, 18

Value in Health Care Act, 47

Value stories: intensive analytics as driver of, 72–74; starting with data, 74–75

Venture capital firms, 4

Virtual care/virtual visits: benefits of, 99, *100*; reimbursement for, 35

Vulnerable populations, 29

Walgreens, 162

Walmart, 75

"Warm handoff," 126

Waste in US healthcare system, six domains of, 111–13; administrative complexity, 111; failure of care coordination, 111, 112, 113; failure of care delivery, 111, 112, 113; fraud and abuse, 111; overtreatment or low-value care, 111, 112, 113; pricing failure, 111

Wearables, 162

Wellness: importance of care retention and, 52; payviders, value-based care, and, 67; population health and global look at, 15; population health management and focus on, 24; programs for, as key element in population health, *16, 17. See also* Community wellness

Whalen, Mark, 52

WHO. *See* World Health Organization (WHO)

Wohlforth, Charles, x

Workforce capability: building, 114

Workforce capacity: stress on, 128–29

World Health Organization (WHO): eight actionable priorities in continuity of care, 113–14, *114,* 123;social drivers of health defined by, 32

Z codes: social determinants of health and, 157

About the Author

Dr. Mark Angelo is the president and CEO of Delaware Valley ACO, a large, payer-agnostic, risk-bearing value-based care organization located in the greater Philadelphia region. In this role, he develops and implements strategy for value-based care, network management, payer relations, care coordination, and other clinical aspects of value-based care for Jefferson Health and Main Line Health Systems. DVACO holds successful risk contracts with multiple payers, including a large, enhanced-track Medicare Shared Savings Program population as well as multiple other commercial and Medicare Advantage programs, serving the Greater Philadelphia and surrounding regions.

Dr. Angelo joined DVACO from Cooper University Health Care, where he served as the CEO of the AllCare Health Alliance ACO and the medical director for population health. At Cooper, he maintained oversight of general internal medicine and family medicine while leading activities for the network of primary care providers surrounding strategy, growth, operations, and innovative models of care delivery.

He has experience with matriculation and participation in alternative payment models such as the Oncology Care Model (OCM), the Comprehensive Primary Care Plus (CPC+) Model, and the Bundled Payments for Care Improvement initiative. Most recently, he has facilitated the movement of DVACO to the Enhanced (highest risk) track with a successful focus on provider engagement, clinical care transformation, and accurate risk capture across a large network.

Dr. Angelo is a practicing palliative medicine physician. He was the founding head of palliative medicine within the MD Anderson Cancer Center at Cooper, where he also founded New Jersey's first ACGME-accredited fellowship in hospice and palliative medicine in New Jersey.

In addition to being a champion for patient experience, Dr. Angelo has led providers to make great strides in physician communication in the ambulatory setting. He is well published and has delivered talks locally, regionally, and nationally on various topics, including population health, palliative medicine, ethics in healthcare, and operational excellence. He is a graduate of Temple University School of Medicine, where he also attended internship and residency. He is board certified in palliative medicine and internal medicine, and he holds a master's degree in healthcare administration.

Dr. Angelo lives in New Jersey with his family. He loves to read, is an avid daily fitness enthusiast, and has a black belt in the martial arts.